THIS Fucking Diet Journal Belongs To :

_____

BEFORE **& After**

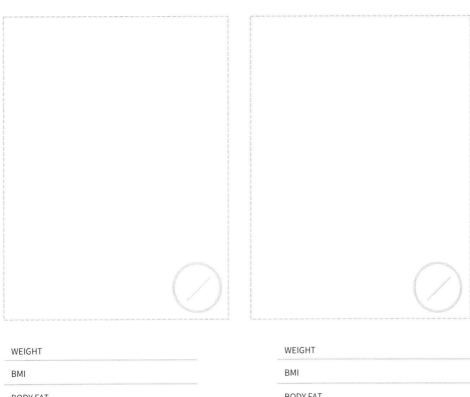

WEIGHT	WEIGHT
BMI	BMI
BODY FAT	BODY FAT
MUSCLE	MUSCLE
CHEST	CHEST
WAIST	WAIST
HIPS	HIPS
THIGHS	THIGHS
CALF	CALF
BICEP	BICEP
OTHER :	OTHER :
OTHER :	OTHER :

WEIGHT LOSS Start Date

My Top 2-3 "WHYs" I Have for Achieving My Most
Fucking Important Health Fitness Goals.

I'm SO Tired of Feeling Shitty – What Fucking Benefits
Do I Want From Following This Diet for 90 Days?

DATE	MY FUCKING WEIGHT LOSS ACTION PLAN		PERSONAL MILESTONES
		☐	
		☐	
		☐	
		☐	
		☐	
		☐	
		☐	
		☐	
		☐	
		☐	
		☐	
		☐	

Health Task Challenge

1 CREATE A JOURNAL AND DOCUMENT YOUR PROGRESS COMPLETED ☐	**2** CHOOSE 7 HEALTHY RECIPES TO TRY COMPLETED ☐	**3** CREATE A WEEKLY MEAL PLANNER COMPLETED ☐
4 LOG EVERYTHING YOU EAT IN A WEIGHT LOSS APP COMPLETED ☐	**5** PURCHASE A FOOD SCALE AND SPIRALIZER COMPLETED ☐	**6** GET OUTSIDE EVERY DAY FOR A WEEK COMPLETED ☐
7 WEIGH YOURSELF EVERY WEEK COMPLETED ☐	**8** GO ALCOHOL FREE FOR ONE WEEK COMPLETED ☐	**9** TRY A 12-HOUR INTERMITTENT FAST COMPLETED ☐
10 CHECK AND LOG YOUR BODY MEASUREMENTS COMPLETED ☐	**11** LIST ALL THE REASONS WHY EATING HEALTHY WILL WORK FOR YOU COMPLETED ☐	**12** STRENGTHEN HEALTHY RELATIONSHIPS WITH OTHERS COMPLETED ☐
13 MONITOR YOUR WATER INTAKE COMPLETED ☐	**14** INCREASE YOUR HEALTHY FAT INTAKE COMPLETED ☐	**15** GET GOOD SLEEP EVERY NIGHT FOR A WEEK COMPLETED ☐

My GO TO **Meals**

HEALTHY MEALS I'D *DIE* FOR (OR MAYBE THEY'RE
JUST SIMPLE TO MAKE)

BREAKFAST	LUNCH	DINNER	SNACKS
BREAKFAST	LUNCH	DINNER	SNACKS
BREAKFAST	LUNCH	DINNER	SNACKS
BREAKFAST	LUNCH	DINNER	SNACKS
BREAKFAST	LUNCH	DINNER	SNACKS
BREAKFAST	LUNCH	DINNER	SNACKS
BREAKFAST	LUNCH	DINNER	SNACKS

WEIGHT LOSS **Tracker**

MONTHLY GOAL

WEEKLY MEASUREMENTS
& WEIGHT LOSS TRACKER
LET'S GET THIS SH*T DONE!!

DATE:

	BUST				
	WAIST				
	HIPS				
	BICEP				
	THIGH				
	CALF				
	WEIGHT				

TOTAL WEIGHT LOSS >>

INTERMITTENT **Fasting Log**

WEEK OF:

	START TIME	END TIME	TOTAL FAST HRS
M	:	:	:
T	:	:	:
W	:	:	:
T	:	:	:
F	:	:	:
S	:	:	:
S	:	:	:

WEEK OF:

	START TIME	END TIME	TOTAL FAST HRS
M	:	:	:
T	:	:	:
W	:	:	:
T	:	:	:
F	:	:	:
S	:	:	:
S	:	:	:

WEEK OF:

	START TIME	END TIME	TOTAL FAST HRS
M	:	:	:
T	:	:	:
W	:	:	:
T	:	:	:
F	:	:	:
S	:	:	:
S	:	:	:

WEEK OF:

	START TIME	END TIME	TOTAL FAST HRS
M	:	:	:
T	:	:	:
W	:	:	:
T	:	:	:
F	:	:	:
S	:	:	:
S	:	:	:

WEEK OF:

	START TIME	END TIME	TOTAL FAST HRS
M	:	:	:
T	:	:	:
W	:	:	:
T	:	:	:
F	:	:	:
S	:	:	:
S	:	:	:

NOTES & REFLECTIONS & SHIT

MILESTONES & ACCOMPLISHMENTS

GOALS &
Accomplishments

MONTH | JAN FEB MAR APR MAY JUN JUL AUG SEP OCT NOV DEC

THIS MONTH'S FUCKING GOALS

MY FUCKING ACTION PLAN

M T W T F S S

☐☐☐☐☐☐☐
☐☐☐☐☐☐☐
☐☐☐☐☐☐☐
☐☐☐☐☐☐☐
☐☐☐☐☐☐☐

NOTES:

WEEKLY GOALS

THOUGHTS

MEAL IDEAS:	BREAKFAST	LUNCH	DINNER	SNACKS
M				
T				
W				
T				
F				
S				
S				

MEAL **Planner**

WEEK OF

GROCERY LIST

MON

TUES

WED

THUR

FRI

SAT

SUN

MY Shopping List

FRESH PRODUCE

MEAT AND SEAFOOD

DAIRY PRODUCTS

PANTRY ITEMS

FROZEN / OTHER

I MAKE PROGRESS **EVERY Day**

SLEEP TRACKER:

DATE

RISE: | BEDTIME: | SLEEP (HRS):

MY NOTES FOR THE DAY

DAILY ENERGY LEVEL		
FUCKING GREAT!	**OKAY**	**SHITTY**

IN A STATE OF KETOSIS?

YES NO UNSURE

WATER INTAKE TRACKER

EXERCISE / WORKOUT ROUTINE

BREAKFAST

FAT: CARBS: PROTEIN: CALORIES:

LUNCH

FAT: CARBS: PROTEIN: CALORIES:

DINNER

FAT: CARBS: PROTEIN: CALORIES:

SNACKS

FAT: CARBS: PROTEIN: CALORIES:

SLAY the DAY! – MY TOP 3 PRIORITIES

-
-
-

END OF THE DAY TOTAL OVERVIEW

FAT CARBS PROTEIN KCAL

I MAKE PROGRESS **EVERY Day**

SLEEP TRACKER: DATE _____

☼ RISE: _____   ☾ᶻᶻᶻ BEDTIME: _____   💭ᶻᶻᶻ SLEEP (HRS): _____

MY NOTES FOR THE DAY

_____

_____

IN A STATE OF KETOSIS?

YES   NO   UNSURE

WATER INTAKE TRACKER

💧 💧 💧 💧 💧 💧 💧 💧

EXERCISE / WORKOUT ROUTINE

SLAY the DAY! – MY TOP 3 PRIORITIES

○ _____

○ _____

○ _____

DAILY ENERGY LEVEL

FUCKING GREAT!   OKAY   SHITTY

BREAKFAST

FAT: CARBS: PROTEIN: CALORIES:

LUNCH

FAT: CARBS: PROTEIN: CALORIES:

DINNER

FAT: CARBS: PROTEIN: CALORIES:

SNACKS

FAT: CARBS: PROTEIN: CALORIES:

END OF THE DAY TOTAL OVERVIEW

FAT	CARBS	PROTEIN	KCAL

I MAKE PROGRESS **EVERY Day**

SLEEP TRACKER:

DATE _____

☼ | RISE: _____

🌙 zᶻᶻ | BEDTIME: _____

💤 | SLEEP (HRS): _____

MY NOTES FOR THE DAY
_____
_____

IN A STATE OF KETOSIS?

YES   NO   UNSURE

WATER INTAKE TRACKER

EXERCISE / WORKOUT ROUTINE

SLAY the DAY! – MY TOP 3 PRIORITIES

○ _____
○ _____
○ _____

DAILY ENERGY LEVEL

FUCKING GREAT!   **OKAY**   **SHITTY**

BREAKFAST

FAT: CARBS: PROTEIN: CALORIES:

LUNCH

FAT: CARBS: PROTEIN: CALORIES:

DINNER

FAT: CARBS: PROTEIN: CALORIES:

SNACKS

FAT: CARBS: PROTEIN: CALORIES:

END OF THE DAY TOTAL OVERVIEW

FAT	CARBS	PROTEIN	KCAL

I MAKE PROGRESS **EVERY Day**

SLEEP TRACKER:

DATE _____

☀ RISE: _____   🌙 BEDTIME: _____   💤 SLEEP (HRS): _____

MY NOTES FOR THE DAY

_____

_____

_____

IN A STATE OF KETOSIS?

YES   NO   UNSURE

WATER INTAKE TRACKER

💧 💧 💧 💧 💧 💧 💧 💧 💧 💧

EXERCISE / WORKOUT ROUTINE

SLAY the DAY! – MY TOP 3 PRIORITIES

● _____

● _____

● _____

DAILY ENERGY LEVEL
FUCKING GREAT!   OKAY   SHITTY

BREAKFAST

FAT: CARBS: PROTEIN: CALORIES:

LUNCH

FAT: CARBS: PROTEIN: CALORIES:

DINNER

FAT: CARBS: PROTEIN: CALORIES:

SNACKS

FAT: CARBS: PROTEIN: CALORIES:

END OF THE DAY TOTAL OVERVIEW

FAT	CARBS	PROTEIN	KCAL
_____	_____	_____	_____

I MAKE PROGRESS **EVERY Day**

SLEEP TRACKER:

RISE: BEDTIME: SLEEP (HRS):

MY NOTES FOR THE DAY

DAILY ENERGY LEVEL

FUCKING GREAT!   **OKAY**   **SHITTY**

IN A STATE OF KETOSIS?

YES   NO   UNSURE

WATER INTAKE TRACKER

EXERCISE / WORKOUT ROUTINE

BREAKFAST

FAT: CARBS: PROTEIN: CALORIES:

LUNCH

FAT: CARBS: PROTEIN: CALORIES:

DINNER

FAT: CARBS: PROTEIN: CALORIES:

SNACKS

FAT: CARBS: PROTEIN: CALORIES:

SLAY the DAY! – MY TOP 3 PRIORITIES

-
-
-

END OF THE DAY TOTAL OVERVIEW

FAT   CARBS   PROTEIN   KCAL

I MAKE PROGRESS **EVERY Day**

SLEEP TRACKER:

DATE _____

☀ RISE: _____ 🌙 ᶻᶻᶻ BEDTIME: _____ 💭ᶻᶻᶻ SLEEP (HRS): _____

MY NOTES FOR THE DAY

_____

_____

IN A STATE OF KETOSIS?

YES   NO   UNSURE

WATER INTAKE TRACKER

💧 💧 💧 💧 💧 💧 💧 💧

EXERCISE / WORKOUT ROUTINE

SLAY the DAY! – MY TOP 3 PRIORITIES

○ _____

○ _____

○ _____

DAILY ENERGY LEVEL

FUCKING GREAT!   **OKAY**   **SHITTY**

BREAKFAST

FAT: CARBS: PROTEIN: CALORIES:

LUNCH

FAT: CARBS: PROTEIN: CALORIES:

DINNER

FAT: CARBS: PROTEIN: CALORIES:

SNACKS

FAT: CARBS: PROTEIN: CALORIES:

END OF THE DAY TOTAL OVERVIEW

FAT	CARBS	PROTEIN	KCAL

I MAKE PROGRESS **EVERY Day**

SLEEP TRACKER:

DATE

RISE:

BEDTIME:

SLEEP (HRS):

MY NOTES FOR THE DAY

DAILY ENERGY LEVEL

FUCKING GREAT!   **OKAY**   **SHITTY**

BREAKFAST

FAT: CARBS: PROTEIN: CALORIES:

IN A STATE OF KETOSIS?

YES   NO   UNSURE

WATER INTAKE TRACKER

LUNCH

FAT: CARBS: PROTEIN: CALORIES:

EXERCISE / WORKOUT ROUTINE

DINNER

FAT: CARBS: PROTEIN: CALORIES:

SNACKS

FAT: CARBS: PROTEIN: CALORIES:

SLAY the DAY! – MY TOP 3 PRIORITIES

-
-
-

END OF THE DAY TOTAL OVERVIEW

FAT	CARBS	PROTEIN	KCAL

I CAN FUCKING
DO THIS

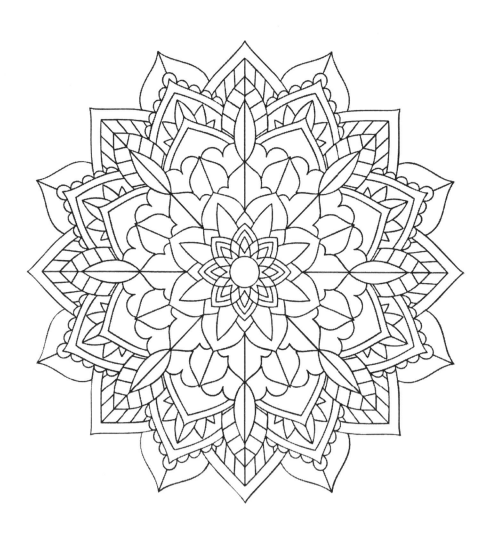

MEAL **Planner**

GROCERY LIST

- [ ]
- [ ]
- [ ]
- [ ]
- [ ]
- [ ]
- [ ]
- [ ]
- [ ]
- [ ]
- [ ]
- [ ]
- [ ]
- [ ]
- [ ]
- [ ]
- [ ]
- [ ]

MON

TUES

WED

THUR

FRI

SAT

SUN

MY Shopping List

FRESH PRODUCE

MEAT AND SEAFOOD

DAIRY PRODUCTS

PANTRY ITEMS

FROZEN / OTHER

I MAKE PROGRESS EVERY Day

SLEEP TRACKER:

DATE _____

RISE: _____ BEDTIME: _____ SLEEP (HRS): _____

MY NOTES FOR THE DAY

_____
_____
_____

IN A STATE OF KETOSIS?

YES   NO   UNSURE

WATER INTAKE TRACKER

EXERCISE / WORKOUT ROUTINE

SLAY the DAY! – MY TOP 3 PRIORITIES

○ _____
○ _____
○ _____

DAILY ENERGY LEVEL

FUCKING GREAT!   OKAY   SHITTY

BREAKFAST

FAT: CARBS: PROTEIN: CALORIES:

LUNCH

FAT: CARBS: PROTEIN: CALORIES:

DINNER

FAT: CARBS: PROTEIN: CALORIES:

SNACKS

FAT: CARBS: PROTEIN: CALORIES:

END OF THE DAY TOTAL OVERVIEW

FAT	CARBS	PROTEIN	KCAL

I MAKE PROGRESS EVERY Day

SLEEP TRACKER:

DATE _____

☀ RISE: _____ 🌙 BEDTIME: _____ 💭 SLEEP (HRS): _____

MY NOTES FOR THE DAY

_____

_____

IN A STATE OF KETOSIS?

YES   NO   UNSURE

WATER INTAKE TRACKER

💧 💧 💧 💧 💧 💧 💧 💧

EXERCISE / WORKOUT ROUTINE

SLAY the DAY! – MY TOP 3 PRIORITIES

● _____

● _____

● _____

DAILY ENERGY LEVEL

FUCKING GREAT!   **OKAY**   **SHITTY**

BREAKFAST

FAT: CARBS: PROTEIN: CALORIES:

LUNCH

FAT: CARBS: PROTEIN: CALORIES:

DINNER

FAT: CARBS: PROTEIN: CALORIES:

SNACKS

FAT: CARBS: PROTEIN: CALORIES:

END OF THE DAY TOTAL OVERVIEW

FAT	CARBS	PROTEIN	KCAL

I MAKE PROGRESS **EVERY Day**

DATE

RISE: BEDTIME: SLEEP (HRS):

MY NOTES FOR THE DAY

DAILY ENERGY LEVEL

FUCKING GREAT! **OKAY** **SHITTY**

IN A STATE OF KETOSIS?

YES NO UNSURE

WATER INTAKE TRACKER

EXERCISE / WORKOUT ROUTINE

BREAKFAST

FAT: CARBS: PROTEIN: CALORIES:

LUNCH

FAT: CARBS: PROTEIN: CALORIES:

DINNER

FAT: CARBS: PROTEIN: CALORIES:

SNACKS

FAT: CARBS: PROTEIN: CALORIES:

SLAY the DAY! – MY TOP 3 PRIORITIES

END OF THE DAY TOTAL OVERVIEW

FAT CARBS PROTEIN KCAL

I MAKE PROGRESS **EVERY** Day

SLEEP TRACKER:

DATE _____

RISE: _____

BEDTIME: _____

SLEEP (HRS): _____

MY NOTES FOR THE DAY

_____

_____

IN A STATE OF KETOSIS?

YES   NO   UNSURE

WATER INTAKE TRACKER

EXERCISE / WORKOUT ROUTINE

SLAY the DAY! – MY TOP 3 PRIORITIES

- _____
- _____
- _____

DAILY ENERGY LEVEL

FUCKING GREAT!   **OKAY**   **SHITTY**

BREAKFAST

FAT: CARBS: PROTEIN: CALORIES:

LUNCH

FAT: CARBS: PROTEIN: CALORIES:

DINNER

FAT: CARBS: PROTEIN: CALORIES:

SNACKS

FAT: CARBS: PROTEIN: CALORIES:

END OF THE DAY TOTAL OVERVIEW

FAT   CARBS   PROTEIN   KCAL

I MAKE PROGRESS EVERY Day

SLEEP TRACKER:

DATE _____

☀ RISE: _____   🌙 zᶻ BEDTIME: _____   💭 SLEEP (HRS): _____

MY NOTES FOR THE DAY

_____

_____

_____

IN A STATE OF KETOSIS?

YES   NO   UNSURE

WATER INTAKE TRACKER

💧 💧 💧 💧 💧 💧 💧 💧

EXERCISE / WORKOUT ROUTINE

SLAY the DAY! – MY TOP 3 PRIORITIES

○ _____

○ _____

○ _____

DAILY ENERGY LEVEL

FUCKING GREAT!   **OKAY**   **SHITTY**

BREAKFAST

FAT: CARBS: PROTEIN: CALORIES:

LUNCH

FAT: CARBS: PROTEIN: CALORIES:

DINNER

FAT: CARBS: PROTEIN: CALORIES:

SNACKS

FAT: CARBS: PROTEIN: CALORIES:

END OF THE DAY TOTAL OVERVIEW

FAT	CARBS	PROTEIN	KCAL

I MAKE PROGRESS **EVERY** Day

SLEEP TRACKER:

DATE _____

☀ RISE: _____   🌙 zzz BEDTIME: _____   💭zzz SLEEP (HRS): _____

MY NOTES FOR THE DAY

_____

_____

_____

IN A STATE OF KETOSIS?

YES   NO   UNSURE

WATER INTAKE TRACKER

💧 💧 💧 💧 💧 💧 💧 💧

EXERCISE / WORKOUT ROUTINE

SLAY the DAY! – MY TOP 3 PRIORITIES

○ _____

○ _____

○ _____

DAILY ENERGY LEVEL

FUCKING GREAT!   **OKAY**   **SHITTY**

BREAKFAST

FAT: CARBS: PROTEIN: CALORIES:

LUNCH

FAT: CARBS: PROTEIN: CALORIES:

DINNER

FAT: CARBS: PROTEIN: CALORIES:

SNACKS

FAT: CARBS: PROTEIN: CALORIES:

END OF THE DAY TOTAL OVERVIEW

FAT	CARBS	PROTEIN	KCAL

I MAKE PROGRESS **EVERY Day**

SLEEP TRACKER:

DATE _____

☀ RISE: _____   🌙 BEDTIME: _____   💤 SLEEP (HRS): _____

MY NOTES FOR THE DAY

_____

_____

IN A STATE OF KETOSIS?

YES   NO   UNSURE

WATER INTAKE TRACKER

💧 💧 💧 💧 💧 💧 💧 💧

EXERCISE / WORKOUT ROUTINE

SLAY the DAY! – MY TOP 3 PRIORITIES

○ _____

○ _____

○ _____

DAILY ENERGY LEVEL

FUCKING GREAT!   **OKAY**   **SHITTY**

BREAKFAST

FAT: CARBS: PROTEIN: CALORIES:

LUNCH

FAT: CARBS: PROTEIN: CALORIES:

DINNER

FAT: CARBS: PROTEIN: CALORIES:

SNACKS

FAT: CARBS: PROTEIN: CALORIES:

END OF THE DAY TOTAL OVERVIEW

FAT	CARBS	PROTEIN	KCAL

ONE DAY AT A FUCKING TIME

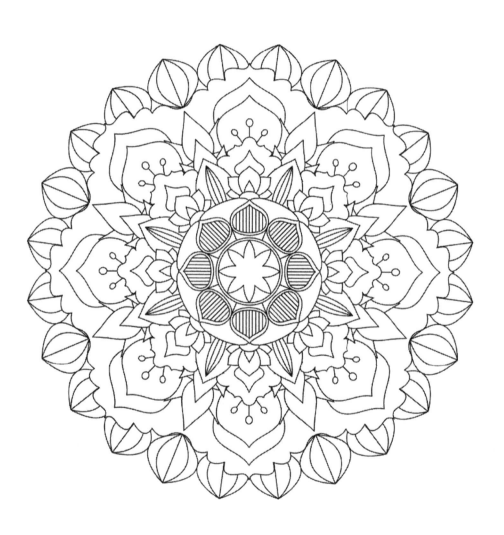

MEAL **Planner**

WEEK OF

GROCERY LIST

	☐
	☐
	☐
	☐
	☐
	☐
	☐
	☐
	☐
	☐
	☐
	☐
	☐
	☐
	☐
	☐
	☐
	☐

MON

TUES

WED

THUR

FRI

SAT

SUN

MY Shopping List

FRESH PRODUCE

MEAT AND SEAFOOD

DAIRY PRODUCTS

PANTRY ITEMS

FROZEN / OTHER

I MAKE PROGRESS **EVERY Day**

SLEEP TRACKER:

DATE _____

☀ RISE: _____   🌙 BEDTIME: _____   💭 SLEEP (HRS): _____

MY NOTES FOR THE DAY

_____

_____

_____

IN A STATE OF KETOSIS?

YES   NO   UNSURE

WATER INTAKE TRACKER

EXERCISE / WORKOUT ROUTINE

SLAY the DAY! – MY TOP 3 PRIORITIES

○ _____

○ _____

○ _____

DAILY ENERGY LEVEL

FUCKING GREAT!   **OKAY**   **SHITTY**

BREAKFAST

FAT: CARBS: PROTEIN: CALORIES:

LUNCH

FAT: CARBS: PROTEIN: CALORIES:

DINNER

FAT: CARBS: PROTEIN: CALORIES:

SNACKS

FAT: CARBS: PROTEIN: CALORIES:

END OF THE DAY TOTAL OVERVIEW

FAT   CARBS   PROTEIN   KCAL

I MAKE PROGRESS **EVERY Day**

SLEEP TRACKER:

DATE _____

☀ RISE: | 🌙 BEDTIME: | 💤 SLEEP (HRS):

MY NOTES FOR THE DAY

_____

_____

IN A STATE OF KETOSIS?

YES   NO   UNSURE

WATER INTAKE TRACKER

💧 💧 💧 💧 💧 💧 💧 💧

EXERCISE / WORKOUT ROUTINE

SLAY the DAY! – MY TOP 3 PRIORITIES

○ _____

○ _____

○ _____

DAILY ENERGY LEVEL

FUCKING GREAT!   **OKAY**   **SHITTY**

BREAKFAST

FAT: CARBS: PROTEIN: CALORIES:

LUNCH

FAT: CARBS: PROTEIN: CALORIES:

DINNER

FAT: CARBS: PROTEIN: CALORIES:

SNACKS

FAT: CARBS: PROTEIN: CALORIES:

END OF THE DAY TOTAL OVERVIEW

FAT	CARBS	PROTEIN	KCAL

I MAKE PROGRESS **EVERY Day**

SLEEP TRACKER:

DATE ....

RISE: ....

BEDTIME: ....

SLEEP (HRS): ....

MY NOTES FOR THE DAY

....

....

....

IN A STATE OF KETOSIS?

YES   NO   UNSURE

WATER INTAKE TRACKER

EXERCISE / WORKOUT ROUTINE

SLAY the DAY! – MY TOP 3 PRIORITIES

- ....
- ....
- ....

DAILY ENERGY LEVEL

FUCKING GREAT!   **OKAY**   **SHITTY**

BREAKFAST

FAT: CARBS: PROTEIN: CALORIES:

LUNCH

FAT: CARBS: PROTEIN: CALORIES:

DINNER

FAT: CARBS: PROTEIN: CALORIES:

SNACKS

FAT: CARBS: PROTEIN: CALORIES:

END OF THE DAY TOTAL OVERVIEW

FAT	CARBS	PROTEIN	KCAL

I MAKE PROGRESS **EVERY** Day

SLEEP TRACKER:

DATE _____

RISE: _____   BEDTIME: _____   SLEEP (HRS): _____

MY NOTES FOR THE DAY

_____

_____

_____

IN A STATE OF KETOSIS?

YES   NO   UNSURE

WATER INTAKE TRACKER

EXERCISE / WORKOUT ROUTINE

SLAY the DAY! – MY TOP 3 PRIORITIES

- ○ _____
- ○ _____
- ○ _____

DAILY ENERGY LEVEL

FUCKING GREAT!   **OKAY**   **SHITTY**

BREAKFAST

FAT: CARBS: PROTEIN: CALORIES:

LUNCH

FAT: CARBS: PROTEIN: CALORIES:

DINNER

FAT: CARBS: PROTEIN: CALORIES:

SNACKS

FAT: CARBS: PROTEIN: CALORIES:

END OF THE DAY TOTAL OVERVIEW

FAT	CARBS	PROTEIN	KCAL

I MAKE PROGRESS **EVERY Day**

SLEEP TRACKER:

DATE _____

☀ RISE: _____ 🌙 BEDTIME: _____ 💭 SLEEP (HRS): _____

MY NOTES FOR THE DAY

_____

_____

_____

IN A STATE OF KETOSIS?

YES   NO   UNSURE

WATER INTAKE TRACKER

💧 💧 💧 💧 💧 💧 💧 💧

EXERCISE / WORKOUT ROUTINE

SLAY the DAY! – MY TOP 3 PRIORITIES

○ _____

○ _____

○ _____

DAILY ENERGY LEVEL

FUCKING GREAT!   **OKAY**   **SHITTY**

BREAKFAST

FAT: CARBS: PROTEIN: CALORIES:

LUNCH

FAT: CARBS: PROTEIN: CALORIES:

DINNER

FAT: CARBS: PROTEIN: CALORIES:

SNACKS

FAT: CARBS: PROTEIN: CALORIES:

END OF THE DAY TOTAL OVERVIEW

FAT	CARBS	PROTEIN	KCAL

I MAKE PROGRESS **EVERY Day**

SLEEP TRACKER:

DATE _____

☀ RISE: _____ 🌙 BEDTIME: _____ 💭 SLEEP (HRS): _____

MY NOTES FOR THE DAY

_____
_____
_____
_____

IN A STATE OF KETOSIS?

YES   NO   UNSURE

WATER INTAKE TRACKER

💧 💧 💧 💧 💧 💧 💧 💧

EXERCISE / WORKOUT ROUTINE

SLAY the DAY! – MY TOP 3 PRIORITIES

○ _____
○ _____
○ _____

DAILY ENERGY LEVEL

FUCKING GREAT!   OKAY   SHITTY

BREAKFAST

FAT: CARBS: PROTEIN: CALORIES:

LUNCH

FAT: CARBS: PROTEIN: CALORIES:

DINNER

FAT: CARBS: PROTEIN: CALORIES:

SNACKS

FAT: CARBS: PROTEIN: CALORIES:

END OF THE DAY TOTAL OVERVIEW

FAT	CARBS	PROTEIN	KCAL

I MAKE PROGRESS **EVERY Day**

SLEEP TRACKER:

DATE

RISE: BEDTIME: SLEEP (HRS):

MY NOTES FOR THE DAY

DAILY ENERGY LEVEL

FUCKING GREAT!   **OKAY**   **SHITTY**

IN A STATE OF KETOSIS?

YES   NO   UNSURE

WATER INTAKE TRACKER

EXERCISE / WORKOUT ROUTINE

BREAKFAST

FAT: CARBS: PROTEIN: CALORIES:

LUNCH

FAT: CARBS: PROTEIN: CALORIES:

DINNER

FAT: CARBS: PROTEIN: CALORIES:

SNACKS

FAT: CARBS: PROTEIN: CALORIES:

SLAY the DAY! – MY TOP 3 PRIORITIES

END OF THE DAY TOTAL OVERVIEW

FAT	CARBS	PROTEIN	KCAL

GET THIS SHIT DONE!

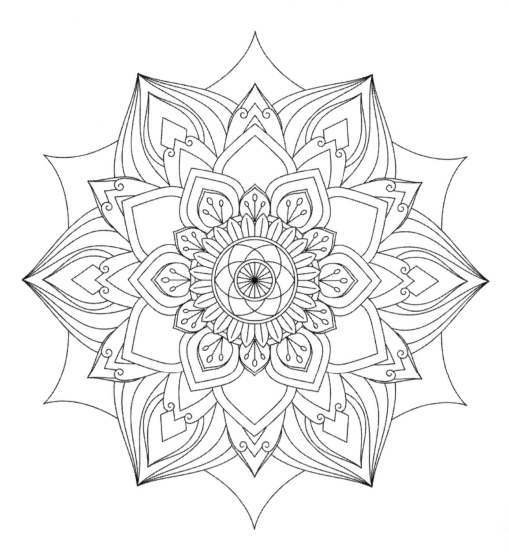

MEAL Planner

GROCERY LIST

- [ ]
- [ ]
- [ ]
- [ ]
- [ ]
- [ ]
- [ ]
- [ ]
- [ ]
- [ ]
- [ ]
- [ ]
- [ ]
- [ ]
- [ ]
- [ ]
- [ ]
- [ ]

MON

TUES

WED

THUR

FRI

SAT

SUN

MY Shopping List

FRESH PRODUCE

MEAT AND SEAFOOD

DAIRY PRODUCTS

PANTRY ITEMS

FROZEN / OTHER

I MAKE PROGRESS **EVERY Day**

SLEEP TRACKER:

DATE _____

☼ RISE: _____   ☾ z z z BEDTIME: _____   💤 SLEEP (HRS): _____

MY NOTES FOR THE DAY

_____

_____

IN A STATE OF KETOSIS?

YES   NO   UNSURE

WATER INTAKE TRACKER

EXERCISE / WORKOUT ROUTINE

SLAY the DAY! – MY TOP 3 PRIORITIES

○ _____

○ _____

○ _____

DAILY ENERGY LEVEL

FUCKING GREAT!   **OKAY**   **SHITTY**

BREAKFAST

FAT: CARBS: PROTEIN: CALORIES:

LUNCH

FAT: CARBS: PROTEIN: CALORIES:

DINNER

FAT: CARBS: PROTEIN: CALORIES:

SNACKS

FAT: CARBS: PROTEIN: CALORIES:

END OF THE DAY TOTAL OVERVIEW

FAT   CARBS   PROTEIN   KCAL

I MAKE PROGRESS **EVERY Day**

SLEEP TRACKER:

DATE _____

RISE: _____   BEDTIME: _____   SLEEP (HRS): _____

MY NOTES FOR THE DAY

_____
_____
_____

IN A STATE OF KETOSIS?

YES   NO   UNSURE

WATER INTAKE TRACKER

EXERCISE / WORKOUT ROUTINE

SLAY the DAY! – MY TOP 3 PRIORITIES

- _____
- _____
- _____

DAILY ENERGY LEVEL

FUCKING GREAT!   **OKAY**   **SHITTY**

BREAKFAST

FAT: CARBS: PROTEIN: CALORIES:

LUNCH

FAT: CARBS: PROTEIN: CALORIES:

DINNER

FAT: CARBS: PROTEIN: CALORIES:

SNACKS

FAT: CARBS: PROTEIN: CALORIES:

END OF THE DAY TOTAL OVERVIEW

FAT   CARBS   PROTEIN   KCAL

I MAKE PROGRESS **EVERY Day**

SLEEP TRACKER:

RISE: _____   BEDTIME: _____   SLEEP (HRS): _____

MY NOTES FOR THE DAY
_____
_____
_____

IN A STATE OF KETOSIS?

YES   NO   UNSURE

WATER INTAKE TRACKER

EXERCISE / WORKOUT ROUTINE

SLAY the DAY! – MY TOP 3 PRIORITIES

- _____
- _____
- _____

DAILY ENERGY LEVEL

FUCKING GREAT!   **OKAY**   **SHITTY**

BREAKFAST

FAT: CARBS: PROTEIN: CALORIES:

LUNCH

FAT: CARBS: PROTEIN: CALORIES:

DINNER

FAT: CARBS: PROTEIN: CALORIES:

SNACKS

FAT: CARBS: PROTEIN: CALORIES:

END OF THE DAY TOTAL OVERVIEW

FAT	CARBS	PROTEIN	KCAL

I MAKE PROGRESS **EVERY** Day

SLEEP TRACKER:

DATE _____

RISE: _____

BEDTIME: _____

SLEEP (HRS): _____

MY NOTES FOR THE DAY

_____
_____
_____
_____

IN A STATE OF KETOSIS?

YES   NO   UNSURE

WATER INTAKE TRACKER

EXERCISE / WORKOUT ROUTINE

SLAY the DAY! – MY TOP 3 PRIORITIES

- _____
- _____
- _____

DAILY ENERGY LEVEL

FUCKING GREAT!   **OKAY**   **SHITTY**

BREAKFAST

FAT: CARBS: PROTEIN: CALORIES:

LUNCH

FAT: CARBS: PROTEIN: CALORIES:

DINNER

FAT: CARBS: PROTEIN: CALORIES:

SNACKS

FAT: CARBS: PROTEIN: CALORIES:

END OF THE DAY TOTAL OVERVIEW

FAT	CARBS	PROTEIN	KCAL

I MAKE PROGRESS **EVERY Day**

SLEEP TRACKER:

DATE

☼ RISE: 🌙 BEDTIME: 💤 SLEEP (HRS):

MY NOTES FOR THE DAY

IN A STATE OF KETOSIS?

YES   NO   UNSURE

WATER INTAKE TRACKER

EXERCISE / WORKOUT ROUTINE

SLAY the DAY! – MY TOP 3 PRIORITIES

-
-
-

DAILY ENERGY LEVEL

FUCKING GREAT!   OKAY   SHITTY

BREAKFAST

FAT: CARBS: PROTEIN: CALORIES:

LUNCH

FAT: CARBS: PROTEIN: CALORIES:

DINNER

FAT: CARBS: PROTEIN: CALORIES:

SNACKS

FAT: CARBS: PROTEIN: CALORIES:

END OF THE DAY TOTAL OVERVIEW

FAT   CARBS   PROTEIN   KCAL

I MAKE PROGRESS **EVERY Day**

SLEEP TRACKER:

DATE _____

RISE: _____

BEDTIME: _____

SLEEP (HRS): _____

MY NOTES FOR THE DAY

_____

_____

_____

IN A STATE OF KETOSIS?

YES   NO   UNSURE

WATER INTAKE TRACKER

EXERCISE / WORKOUT ROUTINE

SLAY the DAY! – MY TOP 3 PRIORITIES

● _____

● _____

● _____

DAILY ENERGY LEVEL

FUCKING GREAT!   **OKAY**   **SHITTY**

BREAKFAST

FAT: CARBS: PROTEIN: CALORIES:

LUNCH

FAT: CARBS: PROTEIN: CALORIES:

DINNER

FAT: CARBS: PROTEIN: CALORIES:

SNACKS

FAT: CARBS: PROTEIN: CALORIES:

END OF THE DAY TOTAL OVERVIEW

FAT	CARBS	PROTEIN	KCAL

I MAKE PROGRESS **EVERY Day**

SLEEP TRACKER:

DATE _____

☀ RISE: _____ 🌙 BEDTIME: _____ 💤 SLEEP (HRS): _____

MY NOTES FOR THE DAY

_____

_____

IN A STATE OF KETOSIS?

YES   NO   UNSURE

WATER INTAKE TRACKER

💧 💧 💧 💧 💧 💧 💧 💧

EXERCISE / WORKOUT ROUTINE

SLAY the DAY! – MY TOP 3 PRIORITIES

○ _____
○ _____
○ _____

DAILY ENERGY LEVEL

FUCKING GREAT!   **OKAY**   **SHITTY**

BREAKFAST

FAT: CARBS: PROTEIN: CALORIES:

LUNCH

FAT: CARBS: PROTEIN: CALORIES:

DINNER

FAT: CARBS: PROTEIN: CALORIES:

SNACKS

FAT: CARBS: PROTEIN: CALORIES:

END OF THE DAY TOTAL OVERVIEW

FAT	CARBS	PROTEIN	KCAL

BE THE FUCKING CHANGE

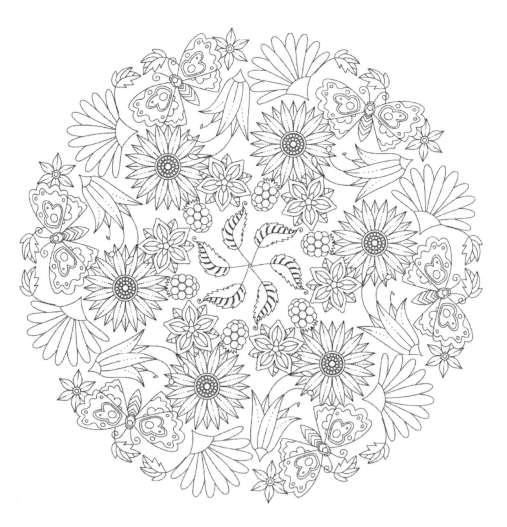

MEAL **Planner**

GROCERY LIST

- ☐
- ☐
- ☐
- ☐
- ☐
- ☐
- ☐
- ☐
- ☐
- ☐
- ☐
- ☐
- ☐
- ☐
- ☐
- ☐
- ☐
- ☐

MON

TUES

WED

THUR

FRI

SAT

SUN

MY Shopping List

FRESH PRODUCE

MEAT AND SEAFOOD

DAIRY PRODUCTS

PANTRY ITEMS

FROZEN / OTHER

I MAKE PROGRESS **EVERY** **Day**

SLEEP TRACKER:

DATE _____

RISE: _____ BEDTIME: _____ SLEEP (HRS): _____

MY NOTES FOR THE DAY

_____

_____

_____

IN A STATE OF KETOSIS?

YES   NO   UNSURE

WATER INTAKE TRACKER

EXERCISE / WORKOUT ROUTINE

SLAY the DAY! – MY TOP 3 PRIORITIES

_____

_____

_____

DAILY ENERGY LEVEL

FUCKING GREAT!   **OKAY**   **SHITTY**

BREAKFAST

FAT: CARBS: PROTEIN: CALORIES:

LUNCH

FAT: CARBS: PROTEIN: CALORIES:

DINNER

FAT: CARBS: PROTEIN: CALORIES:

SNACKS

FAT: CARBS: PROTEIN: CALORIES:

END OF THE DAY TOTAL OVERVIEW

FAT	CARBS	PROTEIN	KCAL

I MAKE PROGRESS **EVERY Day**

DATE

RISE:

BEDTIME:

SLEEP (HRS):

MY NOTES FOR THE DAY

IN A STATE OF KETOSIS?

YES   NO   UNSURE

WATER INTAKE TRACKER

EXERCISE / WORKOUT ROUTINE

SLAY the DAY! – MY TOP 3 PRIORITIES

-
-
-

DAILY ENERGY LEVEL

FUCKING GREAT!   **OKAY**   **SHITTY**

BREAKFAST

FAT: CARBS: PROTEIN: CALORIES:

LUNCH

FAT: CARBS: PROTEIN: CALORIES:

DINNER

FAT: CARBS: PROTEIN: CALORIES:

SNACKS

FAT: CARBS: PROTEIN: CALORIES:

END OF THE DAY TOTAL OVERVIEW

FAT	CARBS	PROTEIN	KCAL

WEIGHT LOSS **Tracker**

MONTHLY GOAL

DATE:

	BUST				
	WAIST				
	HIPS				
	BICEP				
	THIGH				
	CALF				
	WEIGHT				

TOTAL WEIGHT LOSS >>

INTERMITTENT Fasting Log

WEEK OF:

	START TIME	END TIME	TOTAL FAST HRS
M	:	:	:
T	:	:	:
W	:	:	:
T	:	:	:
F	:	:	:
S	:	:	:
S	:	:	:

WEEK OF:

	START TIME	END TIME	TOTAL FAST HRS
M	:	:	:
T	:	:	:
W	:	:	:
T	:	:	:
F	:	:	:
S	:	:	:
S	:	:	:

WEEK OF:

	START TIME	END TIME	TOTAL FAST HRS
M	:	:	:
T	:	:	:
W	:	:	:
T	:	:	:
F	:	:	:
S	:	:	:
S	:	:	:

WEEK OF:

	START TIME	END TIME	TOTAL FAST HRS
M	:	:	:
T	:	:	:
W	:	:	:
T	:	:	:
F	:	:	:
S	:	:	:
S	:	:	:

WEEK OF:

	START TIME	END TIME	TOTAL FAST HRS
M	:	:	:
T	:	:	:
W	:	:	:
T	:	:	:
F	:	:	:
S	:	:	:
S	:	:	:

NOTES & REFLECTIONS & SHIT

MILESTONES & ACCOMPLISHMENTS

GOALS &
Accomplishments

MONTH | JAN FEB MAR APR MAY JUN JUL AUG SEP OCT NOV DEC

THIS MONTH'S FUCKING GOALS

MY FUCKING ACTION PLAN

	M	T	W	T	F	S	S
	☐	☐	☐	☐	☐	☐	☐
	☐	☐	☐	☐	☐	☐	☐
	☐	☐	☐	☐	☐	☐	☐
	☐	☐	☐	☐	☐	☐	☐
	☐	☐	☐	☐	☐	☐	☐

NOTES:

WEEKLY GOALS

THOUGHTS

MEAL IDEAS:	BREAKFAST	LUNCH	DINNER	SNACKS
M				
T				
W				
T				
F				
S				
S				

I MAKE PROGRESS **EVERY Day**

SLEEP TRACKER:

DATE _____

☀ RISE: _____   🌙 ᶻᶻᶻ BEDTIME: _____   💤 SLEEP (HRS): _____

MY NOTES FOR THE DAY

_____

_____

_____

_____

IN A STATE OF KETOSIS?

YES   NO   UNSURE

WATER INTAKE TRACKER

💧 💧 💧 💧 💧 💧 💧 💧

EXERCISE / WORKOUT ROUTINE

SLAY the DAY! – MY TOP 3 PRIORITIES

○ _____

○ _____

○ _____

DAILY ENERGY LEVEL

FUCKING GREAT!   OKAY   SHITTY

BREAKFAST

FAT: CARBS: PROTEIN: CALORIES:

LUNCH

FAT: CARBS: PROTEIN: CALORIES:

DINNER

FAT: CARBS: PROTEIN: CALORIES:

SNACKS

FAT: CARBS: PROTEIN: CALORIES:

END OF THE DAY TOTAL OVERVIEW

FAT	CARBS	PROTEIN	KCAL

I MAKE PROGRESS **EVERY** Day

SLEEP TRACKER:

DATE _____

RISE: _____   BEDTIME: _____   SLEEP (HRS): _____

MY NOTES FOR THE DAY

_____

_____

_____

IN A STATE OF KETOSIS?

YES   NO   UNSURE

WATER INTAKE TRACKER

EXERCISE / WORKOUT ROUTINE

SLAY the DAY! – MY TOP 3 PRIORITIES

○ _____

○ _____

○ _____

DAILY ENERGY LEVEL

FUCKING GREAT!   **OKAY**   **SHITTY**

BREAKFAST

FAT: CARBS: PROTEIN: CALORIES:

LUNCH

FAT: CARBS: PROTEIN: CALORIES:

DINNER

FAT: CARBS: PROTEIN: CALORIES:

SNACKS

FAT: CARBS: PROTEIN: CALORIES:

END OF THE DAY TOTAL OVERVIEW

FAT   CARBS   PROTEIN   KCAL

I MAKE PROGRESS **EVERY Day**

SLEEP TRACKER:

DATE _____

RISE: _____   BEDTIME: _____   SLEEP (HRS): _____

MY NOTES FOR THE DAY

_____

_____

_____

IN A STATE OF KETOSIS?

YES   NO   UNSURE

WATER INTAKE TRACKER

EXERCISE / WORKOUT ROUTINE

SLAY the DAY! – MY TOP 3 PRIORITIES

- _____
- _____
- _____

DAILY ENERGY LEVEL
FUCKING GREAT!   **OKAY**   **SHITTY**

BREAKFAST

FAT: CARBS: PROTEIN: CALORIES:

LUNCH

FAT: CARBS: PROTEIN: CALORIES:

DINNER

FAT: CARBS: PROTEIN: CALORIES:

SNACKS

FAT: CARBS: PROTEIN: CALORIES:

END OF THE DAY TOTAL OVERVIEW

FAT	CARBS	PROTEIN	KCAL

I MAKE PROGRESS **EVERY Day**

SLEEP TRACKER:

DATE _____

☀ RISE: | 🌙 BEDTIME: | 💭 SLEEP (HRS):

MY NOTES FOR THE DAY

_____

_____

_____

IN A STATE OF KETOSIS?

YES   NO   UNSURE

WATER INTAKE TRACKER

EXERCISE / WORKOUT ROUTINE

SLAY the DAY! – MY TOP 3 PRIORITIES

- _____
- _____
- _____

DAILY ENERGY LEVEL

FUCKING GREAT!   **OKAY**   **SHITTY**

BREAKFAST

FAT: CARBS: PROTEIN: CALORIES:

LUNCH

FAT: CARBS: PROTEIN: CALORIES:

DINNER

FAT: CARBS: PROTEIN: CALORIES:

SNACKS

FAT: CARBS: PROTEIN: CALORIES:

END OF THE DAY TOTAL OVERVIEW

FAT   CARBS   PROTEIN   KCAL

I MAKE PROGRESS **EVERY Day**

SLEEP TRACKER:

DATE _____

RISE: _____   BEDTIME: _____   SLEEP (HRS): _____

MY NOTES FOR THE DAY

_____

_____

IN A STATE OF KETOSIS?

YES   NO   UNSURE

WATER INTAKE TRACKER

EXERCISE / WORKOUT ROUTINE

SLAY the DAY! – MY TOP 3 PRIORITIES

- _____
- _____
- _____

DAILY ENERGY LEVEL
FUCKING GREAT!   **OKAY**   **SHITTY**

BREAKFAST

FAT: CARBS: PROTEIN: CALORIES:

LUNCH

FAT: CARBS: PROTEIN: CALORIES:

DINNER

FAT: CARBS: PROTEIN: CALORIES:

SNACKS

FAT: CARBS: PROTEIN: CALORIES:

END OF THE DAY TOTAL OVERVIEW

FAT	CARBS	PROTEIN	KCAL

I SAVE MYSELF

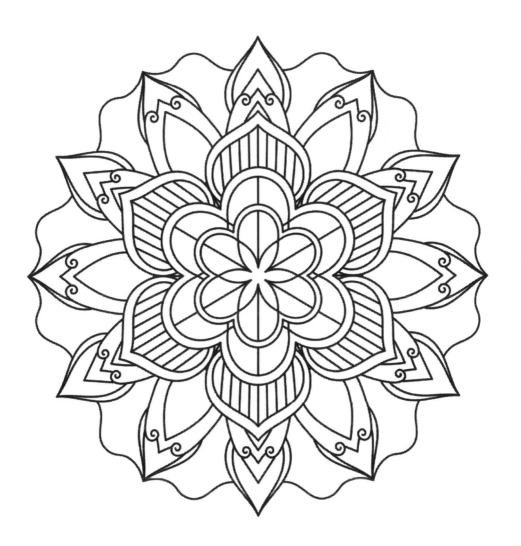

MEAL **Planner**

WEEK OF

GROCERY LIST

- ☐
- ☐
- ☐
- ☐
- ☐
- ☐
- ☐
- ☐
- ☐
- ☐
- ☐
- ☐
- ☐
- ☐
- ☐
- ☐
- ☐
- ☐

MON

TUES

WED

THUR

FRI

SAT

SUN

MY Shopping List

FRESH PRODUCE

MEAT AND SEAFOOD

DAIRY PRODUCTS

PANTRY ITEMS

FROZEN / OTHER

I MAKE PROGRESS EVERY Day

SLEEP TRACKER:

DATE _____

☀ RISE: _____   🌙 BEDTIME: _____   💤 SLEEP (HRS): _____

MY NOTES FOR THE DAY

_____

_____

IN A STATE OF KETOSIS?

YES   NO   UNSURE

WATER INTAKE TRACKER

EXERCISE / WORKOUT ROUTINE

SLAY the DAY! – MY TOP 3 PRIORITIES

○ _____

○ _____

○ _____

DAILY ENERGY LEVEL

FUCKING GREAT!   OKAY   SHITTY

BREAKFAST

FAT: CARBS: PROTEIN: CALORIES:

LUNCH

FAT: CARBS: PROTEIN: CALORIES:

DINNER

FAT: CARBS: PROTEIN: CALORIES:

SNACKS

FAT: CARBS: PROTEIN: CALORIES:

END OF THE DAY TOTAL OVERVIEW

FAT	CARBS	PROTEIN	KCAL

I MAKE PROGRESS EVERY Day

SLEEP TRACKER:

DATE _____

RISE: _____ BEDTIME: _____ SLEEP (HRS): _____

MY NOTES FOR THE DAY

_____

_____

IN A STATE OF KETOSIS?

YES   NO   UNSURE

WATER INTAKE TRACKER

EXERCISE / WORKOUT ROUTINE

SLAY the DAY! – MY TOP 3 PRIORITIES

- ○ _____
- ○ _____
- ○ _____

DAILY ENERGY LEVEL

FUCKING GREAT!   OKAY   SHITTY

BREAKFAST

FAT: CARBS: PROTEIN: CALORIES:

LUNCH

FAT: CARBS: PROTEIN: CALORIES:

DINNER

FAT: CARBS: PROTEIN: CALORIES:

SNACKS

FAT: CARBS: PROTEIN: CALORIES:

END OF THE DAY TOTAL OVERVIEW

FAT	CARBS	PROTEIN	KCAL

I MAKE PROGRESS **EVERY Day**

DATE

RISE: BEDTIME: SLEEP (HRS):

MY NOTES FOR THE DAY

DAILY ENERGY LEVEL

FUCKING GREAT!   **OKAY**   **SHITTY**

IN A STATE OF KETOSIS?

YES   NO   UNSURE

WATER INTAKE TRACKER

EXERCISE / WORKOUT ROUTINE

BREAKFAST

FAT: CARBS: PROTEIN: CALORIES:

LUNCH

FAT: CARBS: PROTEIN: CALORIES:

DINNER

FAT: CARBS: PROTEIN: CALORIES:

SNACKS

FAT: CARBS: PROTEIN: CALORIES:

SLAY the DAY! - MY TOP 3 PRIORITIES

END OF THE DAY TOTAL OVERVIEW

FAT   CARBS   PROTEIN   KCAL

I MAKE PROGRESS EVERY Day

SLEEP TRACKER:

DATE _____

☀ RISE: _____   🌙 BEDTIME: _____   💭 SLEEP (HRS): _____

MY NOTES FOR THE DAY

_____

_____

_____

IN A STATE OF KETOSIS?

YES   NO   UNSURE

WATER INTAKE TRACKER

💧 💧 💧 💧 💧 💧 💧 💧

EXERCISE / WORKOUT ROUTINE

SLAY the DAY! – MY TOP 3 PRIORITIES

● _____

● _____

● _____

DAILY ENERGY LEVEL
FUCKING GREAT!   **OKAY**   **SHITTY**

BREAKFAST

FAT: CARBS: PROTEIN: CALORIES:

LUNCH

FAT: CARBS: PROTEIN: CALORIES:

DINNER

FAT: CARBS: PROTEIN: CALORIES:

SNACKS

FAT: CARBS: PROTEIN: CALORIES:

END OF THE DAY TOTAL OVERVIEW

FAT	CARBS	PROTEIN	KCAL

I MAKE PROGRESS **EVERY Day**

DATE

RISE: BEDTIME: SLEEP (HRS):

MY NOTES FOR THE DAY	DAILY ENERGY LEVEL
	FUCKING GREAT! **OKAY** **SHITTY**

IN A STATE OF KETOSIS?

YES   NO   UNSURE

WATER INTAKE TRACKER

EXERCISE / WORKOUT ROUTINE

BREAKFAST

FAT: CARBS: PROTEIN: CALORIES:

LUNCH

FAT: CARBS: PROTEIN: CALORIES:

DINNER

FAT: CARBS: PROTEIN: CALORIES:

SNACKS

FAT: CARBS: PROTEIN: CALORIES:

SLAY the DAY! – MY TOP 3 PRIORITIES

END OF THE DAY TOTAL OVERVIEW

FAT   CARBS   PROTEIN   KCAL

I MAKE PROGRESS **EVERY Day**

DATE _____

RISE: _____

BEDTIME: _____

SLEEP (HRS): _____

MY NOTES FOR THE DAY

_____

_____

_____

IN A STATE OF KETOSIS?

YES   NO   UNSURE

WATER INTAKE TRACKER

EXERCISE / WORKOUT ROUTINE

SLAY the DAY! – MY TOP 3 PRIORITIES

- _____
- _____
- _____

DAILY ENERGY LEVEL

FUCKING GREAT!   **OKAY**   **SHITTY**

BREAKFAST

FAT: CARBS: PROTEIN: CALORIES:

LUNCH

FAT: CARBS: PROTEIN: CALORIES:

DINNER

FAT: CARBS: PROTEIN: CALORIES:

SNACKS

FAT: CARBS: PROTEIN: CALORIES:

END OF THE DAY TOTAL OVERVIEW

FAT	CARBS	PROTEIN	KCAL

I MAKE PROGRESS **EVERY Day**

SLEEP TRACKER:

DATE _____

RISE: _____   BEDTIME: _____   SLEEP (HRS): _____

MY NOTES FOR THE DAY

_____

_____

IN A STATE OF KETOSIS?

YES   NO   UNSURE

WATER INTAKE TRACKER

EXERCISE / WORKOUT ROUTINE

SLAY the DAY! – MY TOP 3 PRIORITIES

- _____
- _____
- _____

DAILY ENERGY LEVEL

FUCKING GREAT!   **OKAY**   **SHITTY**

BREAKFAST

FAT: CARBS: PROTEIN: CALORIES:

LUNCH

FAT: CARBS: PROTEIN: CALORIES:

DINNER

FAT: CARBS: PROTEIN: CALORIES:

SNACKS

FAT: CARBS: PROTEIN: CALORIES:

END OF THE DAY TOTAL OVERVIEW

FAT	CARBS	PROTEIN	KCAL

WAKE UP. KICK ASS. REPEAT.

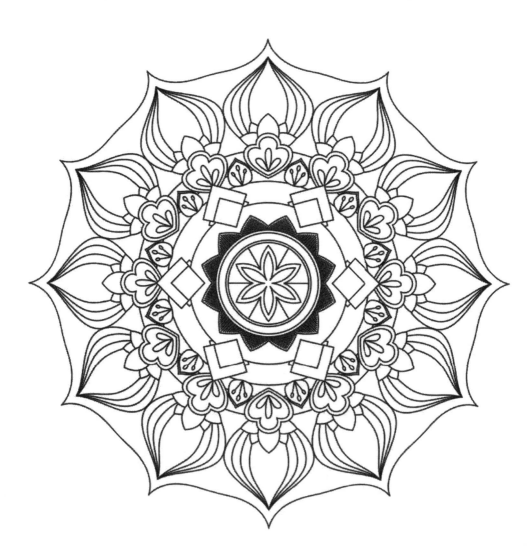

MEAL **Planner**

WEEK OF

GROCERY LIST

- [ ]
- [ ]
- [ ]
- [ ]
- [ ]
- [ ]
- [ ]
- [ ]
- [ ]
- [ ]
- [ ]
- [ ]
- [ ]
- [ ]
- [ ]
- [ ]
- [ ]
- [ ]

MON

TUES

WED

THUR

FRI

SAT

SUN

MY Shopping List

FRESH PRODUCE

MEAT AND SEAFOOD

DAIRY PRODUCTS

PANTRY ITEMS

FROZEN / OTHER

I MAKE PROGRESS **EVERY** Day

SLEEP TRACKER:

DATE _____

RISE: _____

BEDTIME: _____

SLEEP (HRS): _____

MY NOTES FOR THE DAY

_____

_____

_____

IN A STATE OF KETOSIS?

YES   NO   UNSURE

WATER INTAKE TRACKER

EXERCISE / WORKOUT ROUTINE

SLAY the DAY! – MY TOP 3 PRIORITIES

○ _____

○ _____

○ _____

DAILY ENERGY LEVEL

FUCKING GREAT!   **OKAY**   **SHITTY**

BREAKFAST

FAT: CARBS: PROTEIN: CALORIES:

LUNCH

FAT: CARBS: PROTEIN: CALORIES:

DINNER

FAT: CARBS: PROTEIN: CALORIES:

SNACKS

FAT: CARBS: PROTEIN: CALORIES:

END OF THE DAY TOTAL OVERVIEW

FAT	CARBS	PROTEIN	KCAL

I MAKE PROGRESS **EVERY Day**

SLEEP TRACKER:

DATE _____

RISE: _____

BEDTIME: _____

SLEEP (HRS): _____

MY NOTES FOR THE DAY

_____

_____

_____

IN A STATE OF KETOSIS?

YES   NO   UNSURE

WATER INTAKE TRACKER

EXERCISE / WORKOUT ROUTINE

SLAY the DAY! – MY TOP 3 PRIORITIES

- _____
- _____
- _____

DAILY ENERGY LEVEL

FUCKING GREAT!   **OKAY**   **SHITTY**

BREAKFAST

FAT: CARBS: PROTEIN: CALORIES:

LUNCH

FAT: CARBS: PROTEIN: CALORIES:

DINNER

FAT: CARBS: PROTEIN: CALORIES:

SNACKS

FAT: CARBS: PROTEIN: CALORIES:

END OF THE DAY TOTAL OVERVIEW

FAT	CARBS	PROTEIN	KCAL

I MAKE PROGRESS **EVERY Day**

SLEEP TRACKER:

DATE _____

RISE: _____   BEDTIME: _____   SLEEP (HRS): _____

MY NOTES FOR THE DAY

_____

_____

IN A STATE OF KETOSIS?

YES   NO   UNSURE

WATER INTAKE TRACKER

EXERCISE / WORKOUT ROUTINE

SLAY the DAY! – MY TOP 3 PRIORITIES

- _____
- _____
- _____

DAILY ENERGY LEVEL

FUCKING GREAT!   **OKAY**   **SHITTY**

BREAKFAST

FAT: CARBS: PROTEIN: CALORIES:

LUNCH

FAT: CARBS: PROTEIN: CALORIES:

DINNER

FAT: CARBS: PROTEIN: CALORIES:

SNACKS

FAT: CARBS: PROTEIN: CALORIES:

END OF THE DAY TOTAL OVERVIEW

FAT	CARBS	PROTEIN	KCAL

I MAKE PROGRESS **EVERY Day**

SLEEP TRACKER:

DATE _____

☀ RISE: _____   🌙 BEDTIME: _____   💤 SLEEP (HRS): _____

MY NOTES FOR THE DAY

_____
_____
_____
_____

IN A STATE OF KETOSIS?

YES   NO   UNSURE

WATER INTAKE TRACKER

💧 💧 💧 💧 💧 💧 💧 💧

EXERCISE / WORKOUT ROUTINE

SLAY the DAY! – MY TOP 3 PRIORITIES

○ _____
○ _____
○ _____

DAILY ENERGY LEVEL

FUCKING GREAT!   **OKAY**   **SHITTY**

BREAKFAST

FAT: CARBS: PROTEIN: CALORIES:

LUNCH

FAT: CARBS: PROTEIN: CALORIES:

DINNER

FAT: CARBS: PROTEIN: CALORIES:

SNACKS

FAT: CARBS: PROTEIN: CALORIES:

END OF THE DAY TOTAL OVERVIEW

FAT	CARBS	PROTEIN	KCAL

I MAKE PROGRESS **EVERY** Day

SLEEP TRACKER:

DATE

RISE:

BEDTIME:

SLEEP (HRS):

MY NOTES FOR THE DAY

IN A STATE OF KETOSIS?

YES   NO   UNSURE

WATER INTAKE TRACKER

EXERCISE / WORKOUT ROUTINE

SLAY the DAY! – MY TOP 3 PRIORITIES

-
-
-

DAILY ENERGY LEVEL

FUCKING GREAT!   **OKAY**   **SHITTY**

BREAKFAST

FAT: CARBS: PROTEIN: CALORIES:

LUNCH

FAT: CARBS: PROTEIN: CALORIES:

DINNER

FAT: CARBS: PROTEIN: CALORIES:

SNACKS

FAT: CARBS: PROTEIN: CALORIES:

END OF THE DAY TOTAL OVERVIEW

FAT	CARBS	PROTEIN	KCAL

I MAKE PROGRESS EVERY Day

SLEEP TRACKER:

☼ RISE:	🌙 BEDTIME:	☁ SLEEP (HRS):

MY NOTES FOR THE DAY

_____
_____

_____

IN A STATE OF KETOSIS?

YES   NO   UNSURE

WATER INTAKE TRACKER

💧 💧 💧 💧 💧 💧 💧 💧 💧 💧

EXERCISE / WORKOUT ROUTINE

SLAY the DAY! – MY TOP 3 PRIORITIES

- ⦿ _____
- ⦿ _____
- ⦿ _____

DAILY ENERGY LEVEL

FUCKING GREAT!   OKAY   SHITTY

BREAKFAST

FAT: CARBS: PROTEIN: CALORIES:

LUNCH

FAT: CARBS: PROTEIN: CALORIES:

DINNER

FAT: CARBS: PROTEIN: CALORIES:

SNACKS

FAT: CARBS: PROTEIN: CALORIES:

END OF THE DAY TOTAL OVERVIEW

FAT	CARBS	PROTEIN	KCAL

I MAKE PROGRESS **EVERY Day**

DATE _____

RISE: _____ BEDTIME: _____ SLEEP (HRS): _____

MY NOTES FOR THE DAY

IN A STATE OF KETOSIS?

YES   NO   UNSURE

WATER INTAKE TRACKER

EXERCISE / WORKOUT ROUTINE

SLAY the DAY! – MY TOP 3 PRIORITIES

- _____
- _____
- _____

DAILY ENERGY LEVEL

FUCKING GREAT!   **OKAY**   **SHITTY**

BREAKFAST

FAT: CARBS: PROTEIN: CALORIES:

LUNCH

FAT: CARBS: PROTEIN: CALORIES:

DINNER

FAT: CARBS: PROTEIN: CALORIES:

SNACKS

FAT: CARBS: PROTEIN: CALORIES:

END OF THE DAY TOTAL OVERVIEW

FAT	CARBS	PROTEIN	KCAL

I'M STRONGER THAN MY EXCUSES

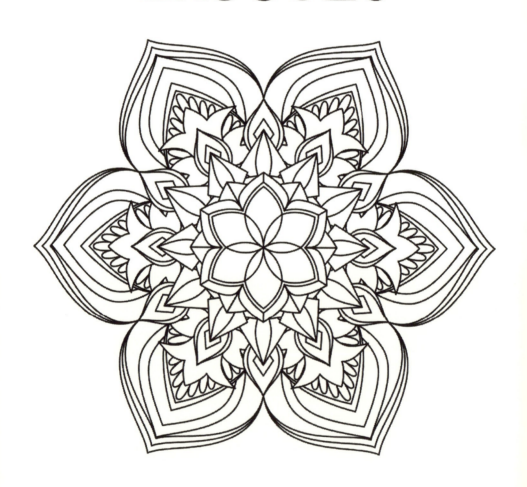

MEAL Planner

WEEK OF

GROCERY LIST

MON

TUES

WED

THUR

FRI

SAT

SUN

MY Shopping List

FRESH PRODUCE

MEAT AND SEAFOOD

DAIRY PRODUCTS

PANTRY ITEMS

FROZEN / OTHER

I MAKE PROGRESS **EVERY Day**

SLEEP TRACKER:

DATE _____

☼ RISE: | ☾ BEDTIME: | 💤 SLEEP (HRS):

MY NOTES FOR THE DAY

_____

_____

IN A STATE OF KETOSIS?

YES   NO   UNSURE

WATER INTAKE TRACKER

💧 💧 💧 💧 💧 💧 💧 💧

EXERCISE / WORKOUT ROUTINE

SLAY the DAY! – MY TOP 3 PRIORITIES

- _____
- _____
- _____

DAILY ENERGY LEVEL

FUCKING GREAT!   OKAY   SHITTY

BREAKFAST

FAT: CARBS: PROTEIN: CALORIES:

LUNCH

FAT: CARBS: PROTEIN: CALORIES:

DINNER

FAT: CARBS: PROTEIN: CALORIES:

SNACKS

FAT: CARBS: PROTEIN: CALORIES:

END OF THE DAY TOTAL OVERVIEW

FAT	CARBS	PROTEIN	KCAL

I MAKE PROGRESS **EVERY Day**

SLEEP TRACKER:

DATE _____

☀ RISE:

🌙 BEDTIME:

💤 SLEEP (HRS):

MY NOTES FOR THE DAY

_____

_____

IN A STATE OF KETOSIS?

YES　　　NO　　　UNSURE

WATER INTAKE TRACKER

EXERCISE / WORKOUT ROUTINE

SLAY the DAY! – MY TOP 3 PRIORITIES

● _____

● _____

● _____

DAILY ENERGY LEVEL

FUCKING GREAT!　　**OKAY**　　**SHITTY**

BREAKFAST

FAT:　　CARBS:　　PROTEIN:　　CALORIES:

LUNCH

FAT:　　CARBS:　　PROTEIN:　　CALORIES:

DINNER

FAT:　　CARBS:　　PROTEIN:　　CALORIES:

SNACKS

FAT:　　CARBS:　　PROTEIN:　　CALORIES:

END OF THE DAY TOTAL OVERVIEW

FAT	CARBS	PROTEIN	KCAL

I MAKE PROGRESS **EVERY Day**

SLEEP TRACKER:

DATE _____

☀ RISE: _____   🌙 BEDTIME: _____   💤 SLEEP (HRS): _____

MY NOTES FOR THE DAY

_____

_____

_____

IN A STATE OF KETOSIS?

YES   NO   UNSURE

WATER INTAKE TRACKER

💧 💧 💧 💧 💧 💧 💧 💧

EXERCISE / WORKOUT ROUTINE

[blank box]

SLAY the DAY! – MY TOP 3 PRIORITIES

○ _____

○ _____

○ _____

DAILY ENERGY LEVEL

FUCKING GREAT!   **OKAY**   **SHITTY**

BREAKFAST

FAT: CARBS: PROTEIN: CALORIES:

LUNCH

FAT: CARBS: PROTEIN: CALORIES:

DINNER

FAT: CARBS: PROTEIN: CALORIES:

SNACKS

FAT: CARBS: PROTEIN: CALORIES:

END OF THE DAY TOTAL OVERVIEW

FAT	CARBS	PROTEIN	KCAL

I MAKE PROGRESS **EVERY Day**

SLEEP TRACKER:

DATE _____

☼ | RISE: |

🌙 ᶻᶻᶻ | BEDTIME: |

💤 | SLEEP (HRS): |

MY NOTES FOR THE DAY

_____

_____

IN A STATE OF KETOSIS?

YES   NO   UNSURE

WATER INTAKE TRACKER

💧 💧 💧 💧 💧 💧 💧 💧

EXERCISE / WORKOUT ROUTINE

SLAY the DAY! – MY TOP 3 PRIORITIES

○ _____

○ _____

○ _____

DAILY ENERGY LEVEL

FUCKING GREAT!   **OKAY**   **SHITTY**

BREAKFAST

FAT: CARBS: PROTEIN: CALORIES:

LUNCH

FAT: CARBS: PROTEIN: CALORIES:

DINNER

FAT: CARBS: PROTEIN: CALORIES:

SNACKS

FAT: CARBS: PROTEIN: CALORIES:

END OF THE DAY TOTAL OVERVIEW

FAT   CARBS   PROTEIN   KCAL

I MAKE PROGRESS **EVERY Day**

SLEEP TRACKER:

DATE

RISE:

BEDTIME:

SLEEP (HRS):

MY NOTES FOR THE DAY

DAILY ENERGY LEVEL

FUCKING GREAT!   **OKAY**   **SHITTY**

IN A STATE OF KETOSIS?

YES   NO   UNSURE

WATER INTAKE TRACKER

EXERCISE / WORKOUT ROUTINE

BREAKFAST

FAT: CARBS: PROTEIN: CALORIES:

LUNCH

FAT: CARBS: PROTEIN: CALORIES:

DINNER

FAT: CARBS: PROTEIN: CALORIES:

SNACKS

FAT: CARBS: PROTEIN: CALORIES:

SLAY the DAY! – MY TOP 3 PRIORITIES

END OF THE DAY TOTAL OVERVIEW

FAT	CARBS	PROTEIN	KCAL

I MAKE PROGRESS **EVERY Day**

SLEEP TRACKER:

DATE _____

RISE: _____

BEDTIME: _____

SLEEP (HRS): _____

MY NOTES FOR THE DAY

_____

_____

IN A STATE OF KETOSIS?

YES   NO   UNSURE

WATER INTAKE TRACKER

EXERCISE / WORKOUT ROUTINE

SLAY the DAY! – MY TOP 3 PRIORITIES

- _____
- _____
- _____

DAILY ENERGY LEVEL

FUCKING GREAT!   **OKAY**   **SHITTY**

BREAKFAST

FAT: CARBS: PROTEIN: CALORIES:

LUNCH

FAT: CARBS: PROTEIN: CALORIES:

DINNER

FAT: CARBS: PROTEIN: CALORIES:

SNACKS

FAT: CARBS: PROTEIN: CALORIES:

END OF THE DAY TOTAL OVERVIEW

FAT   CARBS   PROTEIN   KCAL

I MAKE PROGRESS **EVERY Day**

SLEEP TRACKER:

DATE _____

☀ RISE: _____   🌙 BEDTIME: _____   💤 SLEEP (HRS): _____

MY NOTES FOR THE DAY

IN A STATE OF KETOSIS?

YES   NO   UNSURE

WATER INTAKE TRACKER

💧 💧 💧 💧 💧 💧 💧 💧

EXERCISE / WORKOUT ROUTINE

SLAY the DAY! – MY TOP 3 PRIORITIES

- ⊙ _____
- ⊙ _____
- ⊙ _____

DAILY ENERGY LEVEL

FUCKING GREAT!   OKAY   SHITTY

BREAKFAST

FAT: CARBS: PROTEIN: CALORIES:

LUNCH

FAT: CARBS: PROTEIN: CALORIES:

DINNER

FAT: CARBS: PROTEIN: CALORIES:

SNACKS

FAT: CARBS: PROTEIN: CALORIES:

END OF THE DAY TOTAL OVERVIEW

FAT	CARBS	PROTEIN	KCAL

CAN'T STOP, WON'T STOP.

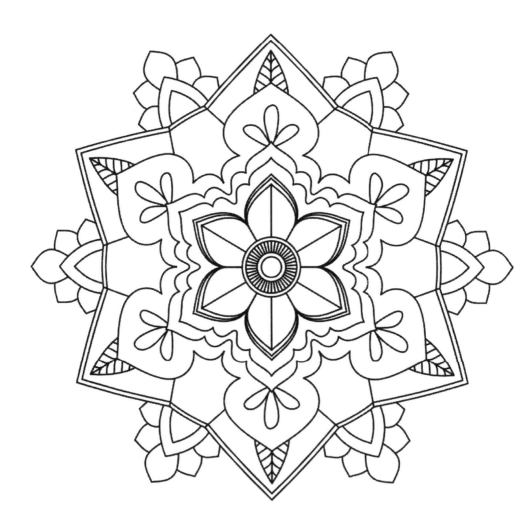

MEAL **Planner**

WEEK OF

GROCERY LIST

- [ ]
- [ ]
- [ ]
- [ ]
- [ ]
- [ ]
- [ ]
- [ ]
- [ ]
- [ ]
- [ ]
- [ ]
- [ ]
- [ ]
- [ ]
- [ ]
- [ ]
- [ ]

MON

TUES

WED

THUR

FRI

SAT

SUN

MY Shopping List

FRESH PRODUCE

MEAT AND SEAFOOD

DAIRY PRODUCTS

PANTRY ITEMS

FROZEN / OTHER

I MAKE PROGRESS **EVERY Day**

SLEEP TRACKER:

DATE _____

☼ | RISE: | 🌙 | BEDTIME: | 💭 | SLEEP (HRS):

MY NOTES FOR THE DAY

_____
_____
_____

IN A STATE OF KETOSIS?

YES   NO   UNSURE

WATER INTAKE TRACKER

EXERCISE / WORKOUT ROUTINE

SLAY the DAY! – MY TOP 3 PRIORITIES

- _____
- _____
- _____

DAILY ENERGY LEVEL

FUCKING GREAT!   **OKAY**   **SHITTY**

BREAKFAST

FAT: CARBS: PROTEIN: CALORIES:

LUNCH

FAT: CARBS: PROTEIN: CALORIES:

DINNER

FAT: CARBS: PROTEIN: CALORIES:

SNACKS

FAT: CARBS: PROTEIN: CALORIES:

END OF THE DAY TOTAL OVERVIEW

FAT	CARBS	PROTEIN	KCAL

I MAKE PROGRESS **EVERY Day**

RISE: _____   BEDTIME: _____   SLEEP (HRS): _____

MY NOTES FOR THE DAY

_____

_____

_____

IN A STATE OF KETOSIS?

YES   NO   UNSURE

WATER INTAKE TRACKER

EXERCISE / WORKOUT ROUTINE

SLAY the DAY! – MY TOP 3 PRIORITIES

○ _____

○ _____

○ _____

DAILY ENERGY LEVEL

FUCKING GREAT!   OKAY   SHITTY

BREAKFAST

FAT: CARBS: PROTEIN: CALORIES:

LUNCH

FAT: CARBS: PROTEIN: CALORIES:

DINNER

FAT: CARBS: PROTEIN: CALORIES:

SNACKS

FAT: CARBS: PROTEIN: CALORIES:

END OF THE DAY TOTAL OVERVIEW

FAT	CARBS	PROTEIN	KCAL

I MAKE PROGRESS **EVERY** Day

SLEEP TRACKER:

DATE _____

☀ RISE: _____ 🌙 BEDTIME: _____ 💤 SLEEP (HRS): _____

MY NOTES FOR THE DAY

IN A STATE OF KETOSIS?

YES   NO   UNSURE

WATER INTAKE TRACKER

EXERCISE / WORKOUT ROUTINE

SLAY the DAY! – MY TOP 3 PRIORITIES

-
-
-

DAILY ENERGY LEVEL
FUCKING GREAT!   **OKAY**   **SHITTY**

BREAKFAST

FAT: CARBS: PROTEIN: CALORIES:

LUNCH

FAT: CARBS: PROTEIN: CALORIES:

DINNER

FAT: CARBS: PROTEIN: CALORIES:

SNACKS

FAT: CARBS: PROTEIN: CALORIES:

END OF THE DAY TOTAL OVERVIEW

FAT	CARBS	PROTEIN	KCAL

I MAKE PROGRESS **EVERY Day**

DATE _____

☀ RISE: _____   🌙 BEDTIME: _____   💤 SLEEP (HRS): _____

MY NOTES FOR THE DAY

_____

_____

IN A STATE OF KETOSIS?

YES   NO   UNSURE

WATER INTAKE TRACKER

💧 💧 💧 💧 💧 💧 💧 💧

EXERCISE / WORKOUT ROUTINE

SLAY the DAY! – MY TOP 3 PRIORITIES

○ _____

○ _____

○ _____

DAILY ENERGY LEVEL
FUCKING GREAT!   **OKAY**   **SHITTY**

BREAKFAST

FAT: CARBS: PROTEIN: CALORIES:

LUNCH

FAT: CARBS: PROTEIN: CALORIES:

DINNER

FAT: CARBS: PROTEIN: CALORIES:

SNACKS

FAT: CARBS: PROTEIN: CALORIES:

END OF THE DAY TOTAL OVERVIEW

FAT   CARBS   PROTEIN   KCAL

_____   _____   _____   _____

[ ]   [ ]   [ ]   [ ]

WEIGHT LOSS **Tracker**

MONTHLY GOAL

WEEKLY MEASUREMENTS
& WEIGHT LOSS TRACKER
LET'S GET THIS SH*T DONE!!

DATE:

	BUST				
	WAIST				
	HIPS				
	BICEP				
	THIGH				
	CALF				
	WEIGHT				

TOTAL WEIGHT LOSS >>

INTERMITTENT **Fasting Log**

	START TIME	END TIME	TOTAL FAST HRS
M	:	:	:
T	:	:	:
W	:	:	:
T	:	:	:
F	:	:	:
S	:	:	:
S	:	:	:

WEEK OF:

	START TIME	END TIME	TOTAL FAST HRS
M	:	:	:
T	:	:	:
W	:	:	:
T	:	:	:
F	:	:	:
S	:	:	:
S	:	:	:

WEEK OF:

	START TIME	END TIME	TOTAL FAST HRS
M	:	:	:
T	:	:	:
W	:	:	:
T	:	:	:
F	:	:	:
S	:	:	:
S	:	:	:

WEEK OF:

	START TIME	END TIME	TOTAL FAST HRS
M	:	:	:
T	:	:	:
W	:	:	:
T	:	:	:
F	:	:	:
S	:	:	:
S	:	:	:

WEEK OF:

	START TIME	END TIME	TOTAL FAST HRS
M	:	:	:
T	:	:	:
W	:	:	:
T	:	:	:
F	:	:	:
S	:	:	:
S	:	:	:

MILESTONES & ACCOMPLISHMENTS

NOTES & REFLECTIONS & SHIT

GOALS &
Accomplishments

THIS MONTH'S FUCKING GOALS

MY FUCKING ACTION PLAN

	M	T	W	T	F	S	S
	☐	☐	☐	☐	☐	☐	☐
	☐	☐	☐	☐	☐	☐	☐
	☐	☐	☐	☐	☐	☐	☐
	☐	☐	☐	☐	☐	☐	☐
	☐	☐	☐	☐	☐	☐	☐

NOTES:

WEEKLY GOALS

THOUGHTS

MEAL IDEAS:	BREAKFAST	LUNCH	DINNER	SNACKS
M				
T				
W				
T				
F				
S				
S				

I MAKE PROGRESS **EVERY** Day

RISE: _____

BEDTIME: _____

SLEEP (HRS): _____

MY NOTES FOR THE DAY

_____

_____

DAILY ENERGY LEVEL
FUCKING GREAT!   **OKAY**   **SHITTY**

IN A STATE OF KETOSIS?

YES   NO   UNSURE

WATER INTAKE TRACKER

EXERCISE / WORKOUT ROUTINE

BREAKFAST

FAT: CARBS: PROTEIN: CALORIES:

LUNCH

FAT: CARBS: PROTEIN: CALORIES:

DINNER

FAT: CARBS: PROTEIN: CALORIES:

SNACKS

FAT: CARBS: PROTEIN: CALORIES:

SLAY the DAY! – MY TOP 3 PRIORITIES

- _____
- _____
- _____

END OF THE DAY TOTAL OVERVIEW

FAT   CARBS   PROTEIN   KCAL

I MAKE PROGRESS **EVERY Day**

SLEEP TRACKER:

DATE _____

☀ RISE: _____ 🌙 BEDTIME: _____ 💤 SLEEP (HRS): _____

MY NOTES FOR THE DAY

_____

_____

IN A STATE OF KETOSIS?

YES   NO   UNSURE

WATER INTAKE TRACKER

💧 💧 💧 💧 💧 💧 💧 💧

EXERCISE / WORKOUT ROUTINE

SLAY the DAY! – MY TOP 3 PRIORITIES

◉ _____

◉ _____

◉ _____

DAILY ENERGY LEVEL

FUCKING GREAT!   OKAY   SHITTY

BREAKFAST

FAT: CARBS: PROTEIN: CALORIES:

LUNCH

FAT: CARBS: PROTEIN: CALORIES:

DINNER

FAT: CARBS: PROTEIN: CALORIES:

SNACKS

FAT: CARBS: PROTEIN: CALORIES:

END OF THE DAY TOTAL OVERVIEW

FAT	CARBS	PROTEIN	KCAL

I MAKE PROGRESS **EVERY Day**

SLEEP TRACKER:

DATE _____

☀ RISE: _____

🌙 BEDTIME: _____

💤 SLEEP (HRS): _____

MY NOTES FOR THE DAY

_____

_____

_____

IN A STATE OF KETOSIS?

YES   NO   UNSURE

WATER INTAKE TRACKER

💧 💧 💧 💧 💧 💧 💧 💧

EXERCISE / WORKOUT ROUTINE

SLAY the DAY! – MY TOP 3 PRIORITIES

● _____

● _____

● _____

DAILY ENERGY LEVEL

FUCKING GREAT!   **OKAY**   **SHITTY**

BREAKFAST

FAT: CARBS: PROTEIN: CALORIES:

LUNCH

FAT: CARBS: PROTEIN: CALORIES:

DINNER

FAT: CARBS: PROTEIN: CALORIES:

SNACKS

FAT: CARBS: PROTEIN: CALORIES:

END OF THE DAY TOTAL OVERVIEW

FAT	CARBS	PROTEIN	KCAL

NO PAIN.
NO GAIN.

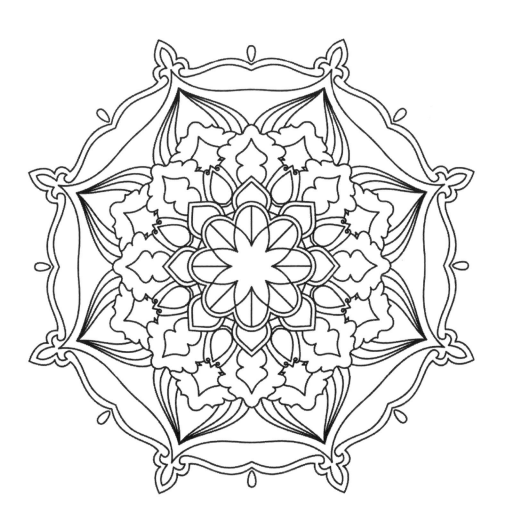

MEAL **Planner**

WEEK OF

GROCERY LIST

- [ ]
- [ ]
- [ ]
- [ ]
- [ ]
- [ ]
- [ ]
- [ ]
- [ ]
- [ ]
- [ ]
- [ ]
- [ ]
- [ ]
- [ ]
- [ ]
- [ ]
- [ ]

MON

TUES

WED

THUR

FRI

SAT

SUN

MY Shopping List

FRESH PRODUCE

MEAT AND SEAFOOD

DAIRY PRODUCTS

PANTRY ITEMS

FROZEN / OTHER

I MAKE PROGRESS **EVERY** Day

SLEEP TRACKER:

DATE _____

☀ RISE: _____   🌙 zᶻᶻ BEDTIME: _____   💤 SLEEP (HRS): _____

MY NOTES FOR THE DAY

_____
_____
_____
_____

IN A STATE OF KETOSIS?

YES   NO   UNSURE

WATER INTAKE TRACKER

💧 💧 💧 💧 💧 💧 💧 💧

EXERCISE / WORKOUT ROUTINE

SLAY the DAY! – MY TOP 3 PRIORITIES

○ _____
○ _____
○ _____

DAILY ENERGY LEVEL

FUCKING GREAT!   OKAY   SHITTY

BREAKFAST

FAT: CARBS: PROTEIN: CALORIES:

LUNCH

FAT: CARBS: PROTEIN: CALORIES:

DINNER

FAT: CARBS: PROTEIN: CALORIES:

SNACKS

FAT: CARBS: PROTEIN: CALORIES:

END OF THE DAY TOTAL OVERVIEW

FAT	CARBS	PROTEIN	KCAL

I MAKE PROGRESS **EVERY Day**

SLEEP TRACKER:

DATE _____

☀ RISE: _____

🌙 BEDTIME: _____

💭 SLEEP (HRS): _____

MY NOTES FOR THE DAY

_____

_____

IN A STATE OF KETOSIS?

YES   NO   UNSURE

WATER INTAKE TRACKER

💧 💧 💧 💧 💧 💧 💧 💧

EXERCISE / WORKOUT ROUTINE

SLAY the DAY! – MY TOP 3 PRIORITIES

● _____

● _____

● _____

DAILY ENERGY LEVEL

FUCKING GREAT!   **OKAY**   **SHITTY**

BREAKFAST

FAT: CARBS: PROTEIN: CALORIES:

LUNCH

FAT: CARBS: PROTEIN: CALORIES:

DINNER

FAT: CARBS: PROTEIN: CALORIES:

SNACKS

FAT: CARBS: PROTEIN: CALORIES:

END OF THE DAY TOTAL OVERVIEW

FAT   CARBS   PROTEIN   KCAL

I MAKE PROGRESS **EVERY Day**

SLEEP TRACKER:

DATE _____

RISE: _____   BEDTIME: _____   SLEEP (HRS): _____

MY NOTES FOR THE DAY

_____

_____

IN A STATE OF KETOSIS?

YES   NO   UNSURE

WATER INTAKE TRACKER

EXERCISE / WORKOUT ROUTINE

SLAY the DAY! – MY TOP 3 PRIORITIES

○ _____

○ _____

○ _____

DAILY ENERGY LEVEL

FUCKING GREAT!   **OKAY**   **SHITTY**

BREAKFAST

FAT: CARBS: PROTEIN: CALORIES:

LUNCH

FAT: CARBS: PROTEIN: CALORIES:

DINNER

FAT: CARBS: PROTEIN: CALORIES:

SNACKS

FAT: CARBS: PROTEIN: CALORIES:

END OF THE DAY TOTAL OVERVIEW

FAT	CARBS	PROTEIN	KCAL

I MAKE PROGRESS EVERY Day

SLEEP TRACKER:

DATE _____

☀ RISE: _____   🌙 BEDTIME: _____   💤 SLEEP (HRS): _____

MY NOTES FOR THE DAY

_____

_____

_____

IN A STATE OF KETOSIS?

YES   NO   UNSURE

WATER INTAKE TRACKER

💧 💧 💧 💧 💧 💧 💧 💧

EXERCISE / WORKOUT ROUTINE

SLAY the DAY! – MY TOP 3 PRIORITIES

○ _____

○ _____

○ _____

DAILY ENERGY LEVEL

FUCKING GREAT!   OKAY   SHITTY

BREAKFAST

FAT: CARBS: PROTEIN: CALORIES:

LUNCH

FAT: CARBS: PROTEIN: CALORIES:

DINNER

FAT: CARBS: PROTEIN: CALORIES:

SNACKS

FAT: CARBS: PROTEIN: CALORIES:

END OF THE DAY TOTAL OVERVIEW

FAT	CARBS	PROTEIN	KCAL

I MAKE PROGRESS **EVERY Day**

SLEEP TRACKER:

DATE ....

☀ RISE: _____ 🌙 BEDTIME: _____ 💭 SLEEP (HRS): _____

MY NOTES FOR THE DAY

_____

_____

IN A STATE OF KETOSIS?

YES   NO   UNSURE

WATER INTAKE TRACKER

💧 💧 💧 💧 💧 💧 💧 💧

EXERCISE / WORKOUT ROUTINE

SLAY the DAY! – MY TOP 3 PRIORITIES

○ _____

○ _____

○ _____

DAILY ENERGY LEVEL
FUCKING GREAT!   OKAY   SHITTY

BREAKFAST

FAT: CARBS: PROTEIN: CALORIES:

LUNCH

FAT: CARBS: PROTEIN: CALORIES:

DINNER

FAT: CARBS: PROTEIN: CALORIES:

SNACKS

FAT: CARBS: PROTEIN: CALORIES:

END OF THE DAY TOTAL OVERVIEW

FAT	CARBS	PROTEIN	KCAL

I MAKE PROGRESS EVERY Day

SLEEP TRACKER:

DATE _____

☼ | RISE: | ☾ᶻᶻᶻ | BEDTIME: | ᶻᶻᶻ | SLEEP (HRS): |

| MY NOTES FOR THE DAY |

....

....

....

| IN A STATE OF KETOSIS? |

YES   NO   UNSURE

| WATER INTAKE TRACKER |

💧 💧 💧 💧 💧 💧 💧 💧

| EXERCISE / WORKOUT ROUTINE |

| SLAY the DAY! – MY TOP 3 PRIORITIES |

● ....

● ....

● ....

| DAILY ENERGY LEVEL |
| **FUCKING GREAT!**   **OKAY**   **SHITTY** |

BREAKFAST

FAT: CARBS: PROTEIN: CALORIES:

LUNCH

FAT: CARBS: PROTEIN: CALORIES:

DINNER

FAT: CARBS: PROTEIN: CALORIES:

SNACKS

FAT: CARBS: PROTEIN: CALORIES:

| END OF THE DAY TOTAL OVERVIEW |

FAT   CARBS   PROTEIN   KCAL

I MAKE PROGRESS **EVERY Day**

SLEEP TRACKER:

DATE _____

RISE: _____

BEDTIME: _____

SLEEP (HRS): _____

MY NOTES FOR THE DAY

_____

_____

IN A STATE OF KETOSIS?

YES   NO   UNSURE

WATER INTAKE TRACKER

EXERCISE / WORKOUT ROUTINE

SLAY the DAY! – MY TOP 3 PRIORITIES

○ _____

○ _____

○ _____

DAILY ENERGY LEVEL

FUCKING GREAT!   **OKAY**   **SHITTY**

BREAKFAST

FAT: CARBS: PROTEIN: CALORIES:

LUNCH

FAT: CARBS: PROTEIN: CALORIES:

DINNER

FAT: CARBS: PROTEIN: CALORIES:

SNACKS

FAT: CARBS: PROTEIN: CALORIES:

END OF THE DAY TOTAL OVERVIEW

FAT	CARBS	PROTEIN	KCAL

SLAY THE FUCKING DAY

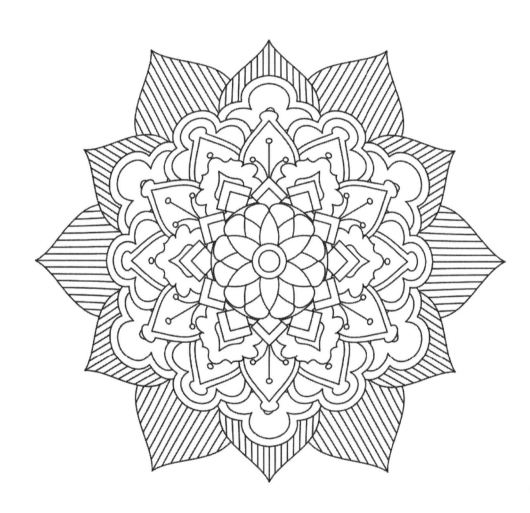

MEAL Planner

GROCERY LIST

- ☐
- ☐
- ☐
- ☐
- ☐
- ☐
- ☐
- ☐
- ☐
- ☐
- ☐
- ☐
- ☐
- ☐
- ☐
- ☐
- ☐
- ☐

MON

TUES

WED

THUR

FRI

SAT

SUN

MY Shopping List

FRESH PRODUCE

MEAT AND SEAFOOD

DAIRY PRODUCTS

PANTRY ITEMS

FROZEN / OTHER

I MAKE PROGRESS **EVERY** Day

SLEEP TRACKER:

DATE _____

RISE: _____   BEDTIME: _____   SLEEP (HRS): _____

MY NOTES FOR THE DAY

_____

_____

_____

IN A STATE OF KETOSIS?

YES   NO   UNSURE

WATER INTAKE TRACKER

EXERCISE / WORKOUT ROUTINE

SLAY the DAY! – MY TOP 3 PRIORITIES

- _____
- _____
- _____

DAILY ENERGY LEVEL

FUCKING GREAT!   **OKAY**   **SHITTY**

BREAKFAST

FAT: CARBS: PROTEIN: CALORIES:

LUNCH

FAT: CARBS: PROTEIN: CALORIES:

DINNER

FAT: CARBS: PROTEIN: CALORIES:

SNACKS

FAT: CARBS: PROTEIN: CALORIES:

END OF THE DAY TOTAL OVERVIEW

FAT	CARBS	PROTEIN	KCAL

I MAKE PROGRESS **EVERY Day**

SLEEP TRACKER:

DATE _____

☀ | RISE: | 🌙 ᶻᶻᶻ | BEDTIME: | ☁ᶻᶻᶻ | SLEEP (HRS):

MY NOTES FOR THE DAY

_____
_____
_____

IN A STATE OF KETOSIS?

YES   NO   UNSURE

WATER INTAKE TRACKER

💧 💧 💧 💧 💧 💧 💧 💧

EXERCISE / WORKOUT ROUTINE

SLAY the DAY! – MY TOP 3 PRIORITIES

○ _____
○ _____
○ _____

DAILY ENERGY LEVEL

FUCKING GREAT!   OKAY   SHITTY

BREAKFAST

FAT: CARBS: PROTEIN: CALORIES:

LUNCH

FAT: CARBS: PROTEIN: CALORIES:

DINNER

FAT: CARBS: PROTEIN: CALORIES:

SNACKS

FAT: CARBS: PROTEIN: CALORIES:

END OF THE DAY TOTAL OVERVIEW

FAT	CARBS	PROTEIN	KCAL

I MAKE PROGRESS **EVERY Day**

SLEEP TRACKER:

DATE _____

☀ RISE: _____   🌙 BEDTIME: _____   💭 SLEEP (HRS): _____

MY NOTES FOR THE DAY

_____

_____

IN A STATE OF KETOSIS?

YES   NO   UNSURE

WATER INTAKE TRACKER

💧 💧 💧 💧 💧 💧 💧 💧

EXERCISE / WORKOUT ROUTINE

SLAY the DAY! – MY TOP 3 PRIORITIES

○ _____

○ _____

○ _____

DAILY ENERGY LEVEL

FUCKING GREAT!   **OKAY**   **SHITTY**

BREAKFAST

FAT: CARBS: PROTEIN: CALORIES:

LUNCH

FAT: CARBS: PROTEIN: CALORIES:

DINNER

FAT: CARBS: PROTEIN: CALORIES:

SNACKS

FAT: CARBS: PROTEIN: CALORIES:

END OF THE DAY TOTAL OVERVIEW

FAT	CARBS	PROTEIN	KCAL

I MAKE PROGRESS **EVERY Day**

RISE: _____

BEDTIME: _____

SLEEP (HRS): _____

MY NOTES FOR THE DAY

_____

_____

_____

IN A STATE OF KETOSIS?

YES   NO   UNSURE

WATER INTAKE TRACKER

EXERCISE / WORKOUT ROUTINE

SLAY the DAY! – MY TOP 3 PRIORITIES

- _____
- _____
- _____

DAILY ENERGY LEVEL

FUCKING GREAT!   **OKAY**   **SHITTY**

BREAKFAST

FAT: CARBS: PROTEIN: CALORIES:

LUNCH

FAT: CARBS: PROTEIN: CALORIES:

DINNER

FAT: CARBS: PROTEIN: CALORIES:

SNACKS

FAT: CARBS: PROTEIN: CALORIES:

END OF THE DAY TOTAL OVERVIEW

FAT   CARBS   PROTEIN   KCAL

I MAKE PROGRESS **EVERY Day**

SLEEP TRACKER:

DATE _____

☼ RISE: _____ 🌙 BEDTIME: _____ 💤 SLEEP (HRS): _____

MY NOTES FOR THE DAY

_____
_____

_____

IN A STATE OF KETOSIS?

YES   NO   UNSURE

WATER INTAKE TRACKER

EXERCISE / WORKOUT ROUTINE

SLAY the DAY! – MY TOP 3 PRIORITIES

○ _____
○ _____
○ _____

DAILY ENERGY LEVEL

FUCKING GREAT!   **OKAY**   **SHITTY**

BREAKFAST

FAT: CARBS: PROTEIN: CALORIES:

LUNCH

FAT: CARBS: PROTEIN: CALORIES:

DINNER

FAT: CARBS: PROTEIN: CALORIES:

SNACKS

FAT: CARBS: PROTEIN: CALORIES:

END OF THE DAY TOTAL OVERVIEW

FAT	CARBS	PROTEIN	KCAL

I MAKE PROGRESS **EVERY Day**

SLEEP TRACKER:

DATE _____

RISE: _____   BEDTIME: _____   SLEEP (HRS): _____

MY NOTES FOR THE DAY

_____

_____

IN A STATE OF KETOSIS?

YES   NO   UNSURE

WATER INTAKE TRACKER

EXERCISE / WORKOUT ROUTINE

SLAY the DAY! – MY TOP 3 PRIORITIES

- _____
- _____
- _____

DAILY ENERGY LEVEL

FUCKING GREAT!   **OKAY**   **SHITTY**

BREAKFAST

FAT: CARBS: PROTEIN: CALORIES:

LUNCH

FAT: CARBS: PROTEIN: CALORIES:

DINNER

FAT: CARBS: PROTEIN: CALORIES:

SNACKS

FAT: CARBS: PROTEIN: CALORIES:

END OF THE DAY TOTAL OVERVIEW

FAT   CARBS   PROTEIN   KCAL

I MAKE PROGRESS **EVERY** Day

SLEEP TRACKER:

DATE _____

☀ RISE: _____

🌙 z z z BEDTIME: _____

💭 z z z SLEEP (HRS): _____

MY NOTES FOR THE DAY

_____
_____
_____
_____

IN A STATE OF KETOSIS?

YES   NO   UNSURE

WATER INTAKE TRACKER

💧 💧 💧 💧 💧 💧 💧 💧

EXERCISE / WORKOUT ROUTINE

SLAY the DAY! – MY TOP 3 PRIORITIES

○ _____
○ _____
○ _____

DAILY ENERGY LEVEL

FUCKING GREAT!   OKAY   SHITTY

BREAKFAST

FAT: CARBS: PROTEIN: CALORIES:

LUNCH

FAT: CARBS: PROTEIN: CALORIES:

DINNER

FAT: CARBS: PROTEIN: CALORIES:

SNACKS

FAT: CARBS: PROTEIN: CALORIES:

END OF THE DAY TOTAL OVERVIEW

FAT	CARBS	PROTEIN	KCAL

GOOD THINGS FUCKING TAKE TIME

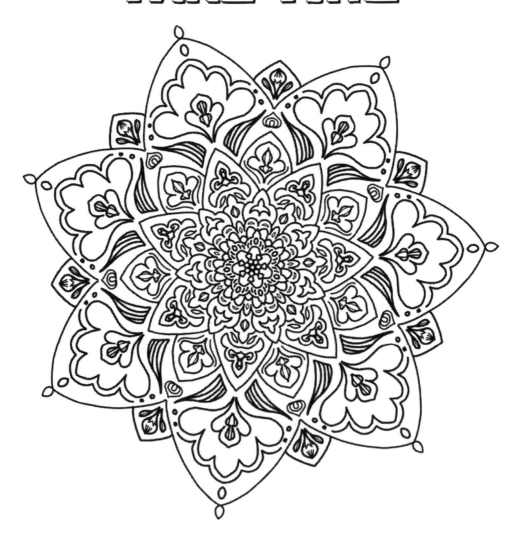

MEAL **Planner**

WEEK OF

GROCERY LIST

	MON
	TUES
	WED
	THUR
	FRI
	SAT
	SUN

MY Shopping List

FRESH PRODUCE

MEAT AND SEAFOOD

DAIRY PRODUCTS

PANTRY ITEMS

FROZEN / OTHER

I MAKE PROGRESS **EVERY Day**

SLEEP TRACKER:

DATE _____

☼ | RISE: | 🌙 | BEDTIME: | 💤 | SLEEP (HRS):

MY NOTES FOR THE DAY

_____

_____

IN A STATE OF KETOSIS?

YES   NO   UNSURE

WATER INTAKE TRACKER

💧 💧 💧 💧 💧 💧 💧 💧

EXERCISE / WORKOUT ROUTINE

SLAY the DAY! – MY TOP 3 PRIORITIES

- _____
- _____
- _____

DAILY ENERGY LEVEL

FUCKING GREAT!   **OKAY**   **SHITTY**

BREAKFAST

FAT: CARBS: PROTEIN: CALORIES:

LUNCH

FAT: CARBS: PROTEIN: CALORIES:

DINNER

FAT: CARBS: PROTEIN: CALORIES:

SNACKS

FAT: CARBS: PROTEIN: CALORIES:

END OF THE DAY TOTAL OVERVIEW

FAT	CARBS	PROTEIN	KCAL

I MAKE PROGRESS **EVERY Day**

SLEEP TRACKER:

DATE _____

☀ | RISE: |
🌙 zᶻᶻ | BEDTIME: |
💭 zᶻᶻ | SLEEP (HRS): |

MY NOTES FOR THE DAY

_____

_____

_____

IN A STATE OF KETOSIS?

YES   NO   UNSURE

WATER INTAKE TRACKER

💧 💧 💧 💧 💧 💧 💧 💧

EXERCISE / WORKOUT ROUTINE

SLAY the DAY! – MY TOP 3 PRIORITIES

○ _____

○ _____

○ _____

DAILY ENERGY LEVEL

FUCKING GREAT!   OKAY   SHITTY

BREAKFAST

FAT: CARBS: PROTEIN: CALORIES:

LUNCH

FAT: CARBS: PROTEIN: CALORIES:

DINNER

FAT: CARBS: PROTEIN: CALORIES:

SNACKS

FAT: CARBS: PROTEIN: CALORIES:

END OF THE DAY TOTAL OVERVIEW

FAT	CARBS	PROTEIN	KCAL

I MAKE PROGRESS **EVERY Day**

SLEEP TRACKER:

DATE _____

☀ RISE: _____   🌙 BEDTIME: _____   💤 SLEEP (HRS): _____

MY NOTES FOR THE DAY

_____

_____

IN A STATE OF KETOSIS?

YES   NO   UNSURE

WATER INTAKE TRACKER

EXERCISE / WORKOUT ROUTINE

SLAY the DAY! – MY TOP 3 PRIORITIES

○ _____

○ _____

○ _____

DAILY ENERGY LEVEL

FUCKING GREAT!   **OKAY**   **SHITTY**

BREAKFAST

FAT: CARBS: PROTEIN: CALORIES:

LUNCH

FAT: CARBS: PROTEIN: CALORIES:

DINNER

FAT: CARBS: PROTEIN: CALORIES:

SNACKS

FAT: CARBS: PROTEIN: CALORIES:

END OF THE DAY TOTAL OVERVIEW

FAT	CARBS	PROTEIN	KCAL

I MAKE PROGRESS **EVERY Day**

SLEEP TRACKER:

DATE _____

☼ RISE: _____

☾z͎ᶻ BEDTIME: _____

☁z͎ᶻ SLEEP (HRS): _____

MY NOTES FOR THE DAY

_____

_____

_____

IN A STATE OF KETOSIS?

YES   NO   UNSURE

WATER INTAKE TRACKER

💧 💧 💧 💧 💧 💧 💧 💧

EXERCISE / WORKOUT ROUTINE

SLAY the DAY! – MY TOP 3 PRIORITIES

○ _____

○ _____

○ _____

DAILY ENERGY LEVEL

FUCKING GREAT!   **OKAY**   **SHITTY**

BREAKFAST

FAT: CARBS: PROTEIN: CALORIES:

LUNCH

FAT: CARBS: PROTEIN: CALORIES:

DINNER

FAT: CARBS: PROTEIN: CALORIES:

SNACKS

FAT: CARBS: PROTEIN: CALORIES:

END OF THE DAY TOTAL OVERVIEW

FAT   CARBS   PROTEIN   KCAL

I MAKE PROGRESS **EVERY** Day

SLEEP TRACKER:

DATE _____

RISE: _____

BEDTIME: _____

SLEEP (HRS): _____

MY NOTES FOR THE DAY

_____

_____

IN A STATE OF KETOSIS?

YES   NO   UNSURE

WATER INTAKE TRACKER

EXERCISE / WORKOUT ROUTINE

SLAY the DAY! – MY TOP 3 PRIORITIES

- _____
- _____
- _____

DAILY ENERGY LEVEL

FUCKING GREAT!   **OKAY**   **SHITTY**

BREAKFAST

FAT: CARBS: PROTEIN: CALORIES:

LUNCH

FAT: CARBS: PROTEIN: CALORIES:

DINNER

FAT: CARBS: PROTEIN: CALORIES:

SNACKS

FAT: CARBS: PROTEIN: CALORIES:

END OF THE DAY TOTAL OVERVIEW

FAT	CARBS	PROTEIN	KCAL

I MAKE PROGRESS **EVERY Day**

SLEEP TRACKER:

DATE _____

☼ RISE: _____

🌙 z_zz BEDTIME: _____

💤 SLEEP (HRS): _____

MY NOTES FOR THE DAY

_____
_____

_____

IN A STATE OF KETOSIS?

YES   NO   UNSURE

WATER INTAKE TRACKER

💧 💧 💧 💧 💧 💧 💧 💧

EXERCISE / WORKOUT ROUTINE

SLAY the DAY! – MY TOP 3 PRIORITIES

○ _____
○ _____
○ _____

DAILY ENERGY LEVEL

FUCKING GREAT!   OKAY   SHITTY

BREAKFAST

FAT: CARBS: PROTEIN: CALORIES:

LUNCH

FAT: CARBS: PROTEIN: CALORIES:

DINNER

FAT: CARBS: PROTEIN: CALORIES:

SNACKS

FAT: CARBS: PROTEIN: CALORIES:

END OF THE DAY TOTAL OVERVIEW

FAT	CARBS	PROTEIN	KCAL

I MAKE PROGRESS **EVERY Day**

SLEEP TRACKER:

DATE _____

☀ RISE: _____   🌙 BEDTIME: _____   💭 SLEEP (HRS): _____

MY NOTES FOR THE DAY
_____
_____
_____

IN A STATE OF KETOSIS?

YES   NO   UNSURE

WATER INTAKE TRACKER

💧 💧 💧 💧 💧 💧 💧 💧

EXERCISE / WORKOUT ROUTINE

SLAY the DAY! – MY TOP 3 PRIORITIES

⬤ _____
⬤ _____
⬤ _____

DAILY ENERGY LEVEL
FUCKING GREAT!   OKAY   SHITTY

BREAKFAST

FAT: CARBS: PROTEIN: CALORIES:

LUNCH

FAT: CARBS: PROTEIN: CALORIES:

DINNER

FAT: CARBS: PROTEIN: CALORIES:

SNACKS

FAT: CARBS: PROTEIN: CALORIES:

END OF THE DAY TOTAL OVERVIEW

FAT	CARBS	PROTEIN	KCAL
_____	_____	_____	_____
☐	☐	☐	☐

DON'T FUCKING GIVE UP

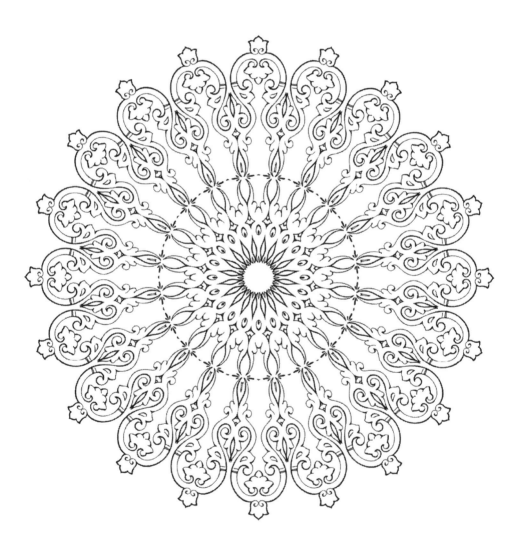

MEAL **Planner**

WEEK OF

GROCERY LIST

MON

TUES

WED

THUR

FRI

SAT

SUN

MY Shopping List

FRESH PRODUCE

MEAT AND SEAFOOD

DAIRY PRODUCTS

PANTRY ITEMS

FROZEN / OTHER

I MAKE PROGRESS **EVERY** Day

SLEEP TRACKER:

DATE _____

☀ RISE: _____   🌙 BEDTIME: _____   💭 SLEEP (HRS): _____

MY NOTES FOR THE DAY

IN A STATE OF KETOSIS?

YES   NO   UNSURE

WATER INTAKE TRACKER

💧 💧 💧 💧 💧 💧 💧 💧

EXERCISE / WORKOUT ROUTINE

SLAY the DAY! – MY TOP 3 PRIORITIES

● _____

● _____

● _____

DAILY ENERGY LEVEL

FUCKING GREAT!   OKAY   SHITTY

BREAKFAST

FAT: CARBS: PROTEIN: CALORIES:

LUNCH

FAT: CARBS: PROTEIN: CALORIES:

DINNER

FAT: CARBS: PROTEIN: CALORIES:

SNACKS

FAT: CARBS: PROTEIN: CALORIES:

END OF THE DAY TOTAL OVERVIEW

FAT	CARBS	PROTEIN	KCAL

I MAKE PROGRESS **EVERY Day**

DATE _____

RISE: _____   BEDTIME: _____   SLEEP (HRS): _____

MY NOTES FOR THE DAY

_____

_____

_____

IN A STATE OF KETOSIS?

YES   NO   UNSURE

WATER INTAKE TRACKER

EXERCISE / WORKOUT ROUTINE

SLAY the DAY! – MY TOP 3 PRIORITIES

○ _____
○ _____
○ _____

DAILY ENERGY LEVEL

FUCKING GREAT!   **OKAY**   **SHITTY**

BREAKFAST

FAT: CARBS: PROTEIN: CALORIES:

LUNCH

FAT: CARBS: PROTEIN: CALORIES:

DINNER

FAT: CARBS: PROTEIN: CALORIES:

SNACKS

FAT: CARBS: PROTEIN: CALORIES:

END OF THE DAY TOTAL OVERVIEW

FAT   CARBS   PROTEIN   KCAL

I MAKE PROGRESS **EVERY** Day

SLEEP TRACKER:

DATE _____

RISE: _____

BEDTIME: _____

SLEEP (HRS): _____

MY NOTES FOR THE DAY

_____

_____

IN A STATE OF KETOSIS?

YES   NO   UNSURE

WATER INTAKE TRACKER

EXERCISE / WORKOUT ROUTINE

SLAY the DAY! – MY TOP 3 PRIORITIES

- _____
- _____
- _____

DAILY ENERGY LEVEL

FUCKING GREAT!   **OKAY**   **SHITTY**

BREAKFAST

FAT: CARBS: PROTEIN: CALORIES:

LUNCH

FAT: CARBS: PROTEIN: CALORIES:

DINNER

FAT: CARBS: PROTEIN: CALORIES:

SNACKS

FAT: CARBS: PROTEIN: CALORIES:

END OF THE DAY TOTAL OVERVIEW

FAT	CARBS	PROTEIN	KCAL

I MAKE PROGRESS EVERY Day

SLEEP TRACKER:

DATE _____

☀ RISE: _____ 🌙 ᶻᶻᶻ BEDTIME: _____ ☁ᶻᶻᶻ SLEEP (HRS): _____

MY NOTES FOR THE DAY

_____

_____

_____

IN A STATE OF KETOSIS?

YES   NO   UNSURE

WATER INTAKE TRACKER

💧 💧 💧 💧 💧 💧 💧 💧 💧

EXERCISE / WORKOUT ROUTINE

SLAY the DAY! – MY TOP 3 PRIORITIES

- ○ _____
- ○ _____
- ○ _____

DAILY ENERGY LEVEL

FUCKING GREAT!   **OKAY**   **SHITTY**

BREAKFAST

FAT: CARBS: PROTEIN: CALORIES:

LUNCH

FAT: CARBS: PROTEIN: CALORIES:

DINNER

FAT: CARBS: PROTEIN: CALORIES:

SNACKS

FAT: CARBS: PROTEIN: CALORIES:

END OF THE DAY TOTAL OVERVIEW

FAT	CARBS	PROTEIN	KCAL

I MAKE PROGRESS **EVERY Day**

SLEEP TRACKER:

DATE _____

☀ RISE: _____   🌙 zᶻᶻ BEDTIME: _____   💭 SLEEP (HRS): _____

MY NOTES FOR THE DAY

_____

_____

IN A STATE OF KETOSIS?

YES   NO   UNSURE

WATER INTAKE TRACKER

💧 💧 💧 💧 💧 💧 💧 💧

EXERCISE / WORKOUT ROUTINE

SLAY the DAY! – MY TOP 3 PRIORITIES

○ _____

○ _____

○ _____

DAILY ENERGY LEVEL

FUCKING GREAT!   **OKAY**   **SHITTY**

BREAKFAST

FAT: CARBS: PROTEIN: CALORIES:

LUNCH

FAT: CARBS: PROTEIN: CALORIES:

DINNER

FAT: CARBS: PROTEIN: CALORIES:

SNACKS

FAT: CARBS: PROTEIN: CALORIES:

END OF THE DAY TOTAL OVERVIEW

FAT	CARBS	PROTEIN	KCAL

I MAKE PROGRESS **EVERY Day**

DATE _____

☼ | RISE: | 🌙 | BEDTIME: | 💤 | SLEEP (HRS): |

MY NOTES FOR THE DAY

_____

_____

_____

IN A STATE OF KETOSIS?

YES   NO   UNSURE

WATER INTAKE TRACKER

💧 💧 💧 💧 💧 💧 💧 💧

EXERCISE / WORKOUT ROUTINE

SLAY the DAY! – MY TOP 3 PRIORITIES

- ○ _____
- ○ _____
- ○ _____

DAILY ENERGY LEVEL

FUCKING GREAT!   **OKAY**   **SHITTY**

BREAKFAST

FAT: CARBS: PROTEIN: CALORIES:

LUNCH

FAT: CARBS: PROTEIN: CALORIES:

DINNER

FAT: CARBS: PROTEIN: CALORIES:

SNACKS

FAT: CARBS: PROTEIN: CALORIES:

END OF THE DAY TOTAL OVERVIEW

FAT	CARBS	PROTEIN	KCAL

I MAKE PROGRESS **EVERY Day**

SLEEP TRACKER:

DATE _____

☀ RISE: _____   🌙 BEDTIME: _____   💤 SLEEP (HRS): _____

MY NOTES FOR THE DAY

_____

_____

_____

IN A STATE OF KETOSIS?

YES   NO   UNSURE

WATER INTAKE TRACKER

💧 💧 💧 💧 💧 💧 💧 💧

EXERCISE / WORKOUT ROUTINE

SLAY the DAY! – MY TOP 3 PRIORITIES

○ _____

○ _____

○ _____

DAILY ENERGY LEVEL
FUCKING GREAT!   **OKAY**   **SHITTY**

BREAKFAST

FAT: CARBS: PROTEIN: CALORIES:

LUNCH

FAT: CARBS: PROTEIN: CALORIES:

DINNER

FAT: CARBS: PROTEIN: CALORIES:

SNACKS

FAT: CARBS: PROTEIN: CALORIES:

END OF THE DAY TOTAL OVERVIEW

FAT	CARBS	PROTEIN	KCAL
_____	_____	_____	_____

SUCK IT UP, BUTTERCUP

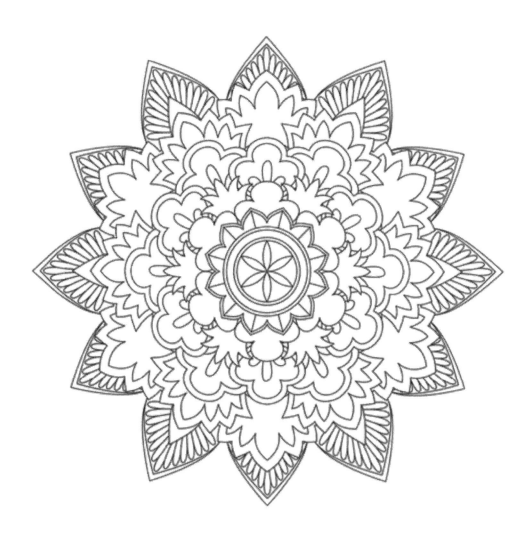

WEIGHT LOSS End Date

*What are some of my thoughts about my
90-Day Journey? How the hell did it go?*

*Will I continue to follow this lifestyle?
What sh*t will I do differently?*

PERSONAL MILESTONES

WEIGHT LOSS **Results**

I FUCKING Finished This Shit!!

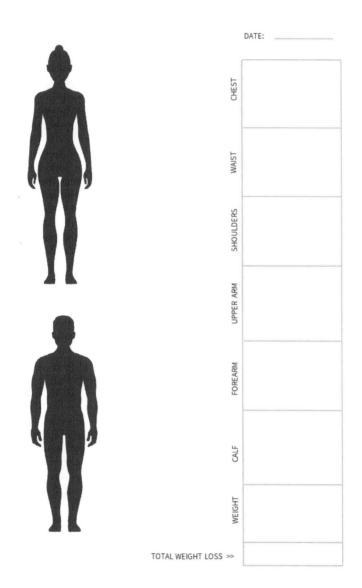

DATE: _____

CHEST	
WAIST	
SHOULDERS	
UPPER ARM	
FOREARM	
CALF	
WEIGHT	

TOTAL WEIGHT LOSS >>

A DAMN GOOD Recipe

RECIPE NAME:

	Keto	Low Carb	Paleo	Vegetarian	Vegan	Dairy Free	Gluten Free
	☐	☐	☐	☐	☐	☐	☐

QTY	INGREDIENTS	RECIPE INSTRUCTIONS

NOTES & RECIPE REVIEW	
	Serves
	Prep Time
	Cook Time
	Tools
	Temp

Total	Carbs	Fat	Protein	Cals

A DAMN GOOD **Recipe**

RECIPE NAME:

	Keto	Low Carb	Paleo	Vegetarian	Vegan	Dairy Free	Gluten Free
	☐	☐	☐	☐	☐	☐	☐

QTY	INGREDIENTS	RECIPE INSTRUCTIONS

NOTES & RECIPE REVIEW

Serves	
Prep Time	
Cook Time	
Tools	
Temp	

Total	Carbs	Fat	Protein	Cals

A DAMN GOOD Recipe

RECIPE NAME:

Keto	Low Carb	Paleo	Vegetarian	Vegan	Dairy Free	Gluten Free
☐	☐	☐	☐	☐	☐	☐

QTY	INGREDIENTS	RECIPE INSTRUCTIONS

NOTES & RECIPE REVIEW

Serves	
Prep Time	
Cook Time	
Tools	
Temp	

Total	Carbs	Fat	Protein	Cals

A DAMN GOOD Recipe

RECIPE NAME:

Keto	Low Carb	Paleo	Vegetarian	Vegan	Dairy Free	Gluten Free
☐	☐	☐	☐	☐	☐	☐

QTY	INGREDIENTS	RECIPE INSTRUCTIONS

NOTES & RECIPE REVIEW

Serves	
Prep Time	
Cook Time	
Tools	
Temp	

Total	Carbs	Fat	Protein	Cals

A DAMN GOOD Recipe

RECIPE NAME:

Keto	Low Carb	Paleo	Vegetarian	Vegan	Dairy Free	Gluten Free
☐	☐	☐	☐	☐	☐	☐

QTY	INGREDIENTS	RECIPE INSTRUCTIONS

NOTES & RECIPE REVIEW		Serves	
		Prep Time	
		Cook Time	
		Tools	
		Temp	

Total	Carbs	Fat	Protein	Cals

A DAMN GOOD Recipe

RECIPE NAME: _____

Keto	Low Carb	Paleo	Vegetarian	Vegan	Dairy Free	Gluten Free
☐	☐	☐	☐	☐	☐	☐

QTY	INGREDIENTS

RECIPE INSTRUCTIONS

NOTES & RECIPE REVIEW

Serves	
Prep Time	
Cook Time	
Tools	
Temp	

Total	Carbs	Fat	Protein	Cals

A DAMN GOOD **Recipe**

RECIPE NAME:

	Keto	Low Carb	Paleo	Vegetarian	Vegan	Dairy Free	Gluten Free
	☐	☐	☐	☐	☐	☐	☐

QTY	INGREDIENTS	RECIPE INSTRUCTIONS

NOTES & RECIPE REVIEW

Serves	
Prep Time	
Cook Time	
Tools	
Temp	

Total	Carbs	Fat	Protein	Cals

A DAMN GOOD **Recipe**

RECIPE NAME:

	Keto	Low Carb	Paleo	Vegetarian	Vegan	Dairy Free	Gluten Free
	☐	☐	☐	☐	☐	☐	☐

QTY	INGREDIENTS	RECIPE INSTRUCTIONS

NOTES & RECIPE REVIEW		Serves	
		Prep Time	
		Cook Time	
		Tools	
		Temp	

Total	Carbs	Fat	Protein	Cals

A DAMN GOOD Recipe

RECIPE NAME:

	Keto	Low Carb	Paleo	Vegetarian	Vegan	Dairy Free	Gluten Free
	☐	☐	☐	☐	☐	☐	☐

QTY	INGREDIENTS	RECIPE INSTRUCTIONS

NOTES & RECIPE REVIEW

Serves	
Prep Time	
Cook Time	
Tools	
Temp	

	Carbs	Fat	Protein	Cals
Total				

A DAMN GOOD **Recipe**

RECIPE NAME:

	Keto	Low Carb	Paleo	Vegetarian	Vegan	Dairy Free	Gluten Free
	☐	☐	☐	☐	☐	☐	☐

QTY	INGREDIENTS	RECIPE INSTRUCTIONS

NOTES & RECIPE REVIEW		Serves	
		Prep Time	
		Cook Time	
		Tools	
		Temp	

Total	Carbs	Fat	Protein	Cals

Made in the USA
Monee, IL
28 March 2020